EVOLVING HEALTH

Maximize Your Energy Using the Wisdom of Science and Divine Design

RUBEN J GUZMAN, MPH

Cover & Book Design by: Aaron Guzman
aaron@coachruben.com

Published 2011
Printed in the United States

ISBN-13: 978-0615487434
ISBN-10: 0615487432

Library of Congress Registration Number: TXu 1-754-788
May 10, 2011

FIRST EDITION

www.CoachRuben.com
Email: info@coachruben.com

Dedicated to all the pioneers who came before me that share my commitment to ending chronic disease on the face of the planet.

CONTENTS

PART TWO: Shifting the Actions and Behaviors

PART THREE: Sustaining the Shifts in Mindset and Behavior

ACKNOWLEDGMENTS

There is probably no way that I can acknowledge everyone who has been a contribution to this book, but I will at least attempt to recognize some of the most significant contributors.

Since this is a transformational approach to health, I would like to thank all my transformational teachers – those who instilled a profound and lasting change in my life. Coach John Wooden who coached the UCLA Bruins to ten national championships in basketball – his pyramid of success and his life have been an inspiration to me most of my life. All my wonderful coaches who showed me the path towards becoming a better athlete and a better person: Jim Rohn, Leo Buscaglia, Denis Waitley, Don Miguel Ruiz, Deepak Chopra, Dr. Wayne Dyer, Jack Canfield, Zig Ziglar, Tony Robbins, Landmark Education and many others.

I would like to acknowledge the following authors whose writings contributed to this book. Lynn Twist, T. Harv Eker,

John McDougall, M.D. (I've been a fan for over 25 years), T. Collin Campbell, Ph.D., Caldwell Esselstyn, M.D., Neil Barnard, M.D., Dean Ornish, M.D., Robert S. Eliot, M.D., Covert Bailey, Ph.D., Stephen Covey, and Leo Babauta.

I am so grateful for the training I received through the UCLA School of Public Health, UC Davis School of Medicine, and the National Academy of Sports Medicine. I am especially grateful to Sorrell Glover, M.D. who was the senior pathologist at Los Robles Regional Medical Center and took me under his wing and mentored me.

Many thanks to all my swimmers, especially Jon Piland, Amanda Horrocks and all my clients. Your courage has been a demonstration of the power of transformation and what is possible.

I wish to thank Brianna Mitchell for her contribution as a clinical hypnotherapist to participants in my program. Many thanks to Amy Brashears, my transcriptionist, and to my son, Aaron Guzman, my producer who did the cover and book design – your help has been invaluable. I am also grateful to my minister, Reverend Kevin Ross, for his support in launching this project.

And, I thank God for everything. Thank you God, thank you God, thank you God!

FORWARD

John Early, Entrepreneur, Board member at Christ Unity Church, Sacramento:

"I applaud you for being here and I want you to know about Ruben's work. Back in September 2009, I decided to do this program because I didn't like the way I looked. I didn't like the way I felt. I didn't like the way my clothes fit on me and a bunch of other things. So, what I did was I made a goal to look like Ruben, and I told him that I wanted to look like him! The other thing I discovered was that I had the goal, but I also needed to have the commitment. Because if you don't have the commitment, forget it! I'm a pretty blunt person on this kind of stuff. This has to be a fun thing for you. So, if it's not going to be fun for you, don't do it, because you won't. If you want to change how you look and how you feel - and it's different for everybody - then get on the program, read the books, get the right food and commit to yourself and just do it. I went out the very next day and got rid of all the food I had just purchased two days before. And the next day after that, I came to him and said there's one food item that I don't want to throw away, I just want to go through and use it. So he looked at me, and he said, "What's your goal, and what are you committed to?" And that's all it took! I got rid of it! So, I encourage everyone to really take this into your heart. And, if you're thinking about it from your head, forget it. Just get up and walk out now. This is life-changing for me and for anybody else who wants to do this. You will not find another program like this. There are other programs that help you to lose weight for instance, but those programs don't take into consideration how your mind works, how we sabotage ourselves, the food that we consume, where it comes from, how it works in your body or any of those considerations. And, this is important. So now, my pants don't fit me anymore, and if I didn't have my belt on they would fall down. I'm not done losing weight. I'm not done reducing or eliminating. So, listen. Listen. Do this program!"

MY STORY

In 1981 I had a couple of experiences that would help establish a foundation for my path in health and fitness. I was a pathologist's assistant, working at Los Robles Regional Medical Center in Thousand Oaks, in Southern California. I had graduated from college the year before, was busy working and also was preparing to enter medical school.

A couple of weeks after I had recovered from a bout of mononucleosis, I began noticing that I was having a pattern of great gastrointestinal difficulty with mild diarrhea every morning, but only in the morning. I had no other symptoms such as fever or anything else, but I was beginning to get a little tired of the inconvenience and discomfort. So, after a couple of weeks of this difficulty, I asked Doctor Glover, the senior pathologist, if he could help me understand my problem. He asked me several questions which seemed inconsequential. But then, he started asking me about what I ate. I explained what I ate for breakfast, and he nodded and said "ahmm." Then I explained what I usually ate for lunch, and he nodded and said "ahmm." I explained what I usually ate for dinner, and he nodded and said "ahmm." Then he asked me if there was anything else...to which I replied that I usually had a bowl of ice cream before retiring for the evening. In response, he raised his eyebrows and said "aha!" He then proceeded to explain to me that I was probably lactose intolerant and that I should eliminate the ice cream from my diet. "Not my ice cream!" I rebelled. So, reluctantly, I complied. But then I noticed that my symptoms also disappeared! And so began my education in nutrition – with a direct appreciation of the relationship between nutrition and health.

One of the duties of my job was assisting in performing autopsies. I realize it may not sound so glamorous or appealing, but I assure you it was an absolutely powerful education. I learned so much about HOW people live since the evidence is quite apparent when they die. One case will remain indelibly etched in my mind. It was the autopsy of a woman in her mid-seventies. She had come to the hospital and died very soon thereafter. What was so unusual about this woman was the condition of her body. She appeared completely healthy – very different from the usual cases. As we began to evaluate her internal organs, we were surprised even further. Her internal organs were as pristine as those of a newborn child! Doctor Glover had never seen such a case. It was truly an amazing sight. It was discovered that the woman's death was caused by a very rare undiagnosed heart defect that in most cases would rarely allow those who had this defect to live past the age of twenty. Why, then, was this woman able to live far beyond the norm? How had she beat the odds? We later discovered that she was a Seventh Day Adventist, one of the longest living groups of people on the planet. The answer seemed to be in HOW she lived – walking five miles a day, eating a vegetarian diet, and taking great care of her body. And so began my education in health and fitness – seeing a powerful example of how to beat the odds.

Another key observation I made from all the autopsies was as a result of a "special" responsibility I had as part of my duties. I know this may sound a little gross, but one of my responsibilities was to dissect the entire gastrointestinal tract and prepare it for the pathologist to examine and take sections for histologic (microscopic) examination, which we did of every organ. Why was this gross, you ask? Well, I basically had to take the entire length of the intestinal tract – 14 to 17 feet – put it in a wash basin, and under running water, I would split open the entire tract and clean it out by hand. Since most of the autopsies were on people who had died of some chronic illness, I noticed something in common with nearly all of them. They nearly all had intestinal tracts that looked, felt and smelled very different from the woman who was a Seventh Day Adventist. These people had intestinal tracts that had much thinner muscular walls. The internal lining was often slimy and mucoid, and lacked much of the folds (rugae) of a healthy tract. It was usually sticky and difficult to clean out. Much of the chyme (food in the digestive tract) that consisted of meat was undigested, since meat doesn't really break down in the intestinal tract – it just putrifies. Therefore, the smell was awful. If you weren't ready for it, the smell would easily make you throw up. All these cases were very different from that of the Seventh Day Adventist. Her intestinal tract had thick, healthy muscular walls. The lining had all the folds of a healthy tract and the contents cleaned out very easily. And, the smell was almost insignificant, comparatively speaking. I truly got to see first hand that we are what we eat, and the evidence was clear in the end.

But it wasn't enough for me to just know how to eat and keep the body healthy and fit. I would have to go through the experience of having to regain health and fitness... for myself. In October 1990 I ruptured my Achilles tendon while engaged in my favorite activity – playing basketball. After the surgery, my physician told me that I should hang up the shoes and that I would never be able to play basketball again without risk of rupturing the tendon again. Of course, I believed him, and thus began an incredible state of depression. For me, not being able to play basketball was depriving me of an important part of my life. For the next four years, I put my head in the toilet and my eating habits went out the window. Before I realized it, I had gained over fifty pounds! Then the day of reckoning happened. I looked at myself in the mirror and said "ENOUGH!!!" I had made a solemn promise to myself a long time before that I would never let myself get overweight like my father had done. Now it was time to re-commit to that promise. And so, I took action. I knew what to do, but knowing makes no difference – I just had to do it. Well, after about a year, I completely lost all the fat and weighed the same that I had when I was a senior in high school, on the basketball and swimming teams. By the way, I now play basketball!

My three years of education in medical school at U.C. Davis were incredibly valuable. I learned so much about the anatomy, physiology, biochemistry and pathology of the body. I also learned that most chronic disease is totally preventable, and that I really did not want to treat sick people with pharmaceutical drugs. My independent research led me to then pursue a Master's degree in Public Health at U.C.L.A., specializing in Behavioral Sciences and Health Education/ Promotion. Then, after working nearly ten years in healthcare administration, I took a break from the corporate setting and lost my weight. I then worked for several years as a clinical exercise specialist and personal trainer, training people to live healthier lives by strengthening their bodies and improving their nutrition. It was by doing this work that I came to realize that my passion is to continue to help people lead healthier and happier lives. I had conducted health education programs related to health and fitness for nearly twenty years. Now, I am committed to bringing my message to the world.

What I have to share with you in these chapters is a transformational approach to attaining optimal health, energy and vitality. I have compiled information that I not only believe, but have also tested... not only on myself, but with countless clients and seminar participants who have embraced my instruction. However, I encourage you NOT to believe everything you hear or read. God knows, there is a tremendous amount of misinformation out there, and a lot of it has to do with just one thing - your money. I invite you to consider what I have to present with a completely open mind. Some of this you may quite readily agree with. Other things will be questionable to you. Yet some things will seem quite revolutionary. Just stay open-minded and consider that this information has already proven itself many times. And maybe, some of it may work for you. So relax, and enjoy the journey. And, thank you for letting me share my ideas with you.

Ruben J. Guzman, M.P.H.

PREFACE

This book is not for those who are hopeful for yet another possible solution to an unending string of failures to lose weight or get healthy. This book is not for those who are still undecided as to whether or not they can commit to making the lifestyle changes that are needed to turn their health around. This book is not for those who are interested in "trying" yet another option.

In the words of Yoda – "There is no try. There is only do."

This book is for those of you who are clear that "This is it! No more!" No longer will you accept defeat. No longer will you accept failure. No longer will you be a victim of what you can't even figure out.

This book is for those who are ready to evolve to a higher level, a higher vibration – a higher lifestyle. This is for those ready to commit to making a profound and lasting difference in their lives, not just a little bit better. This book is for those who recognize that there is a higher power that they need to tap into and they just don't know how to do it. This book is for those who are ready to turn their lives around in a whole new direction, no matter how scary the proposition may seem. If you're ready to commit, then this is the book for you. "For the moment one definitely commits oneself, then Providence moves also."

If you are unwilling to commit, and I mean 100% commit, then don't read this book. Pass this up for now and come back to it when you are ready. But, if you are ready, then buckle up and hold on tight. Get ready to go for a ride that will forever alter the way you live your life, your health, your energy, your vitality – everything.

Don't say I didn't warn you! Now, let's go!

INTRODUCTION

Let's get started. We have a lot to cover. I just want to start by saying welcome to you. Welcome and thank you. I want to also say that I acknowledge you. You inspire me - just so you know. You inspire me because I know it takes courage to take on transforming your health - transforming your body. It takes courage to do that. You could be doing something different right now, couldn't you? Easily! But you're here, and that's out of your commitment to yourself, your health, your vitality. And there's even a ripple effect to that, because there is a commitment to your family - there is a commitment to your work — there is a commitment to your passions — there's a commitment to your communities. You being on this planet... I mean it's part of one of the things about John that really inspired me is that he realized for himself, that he has a profound mission of what he needs to be able to do while he is on this planet. He wants to be able to live long enough to fulfill his mission. He was realizing he was going to a place where he wasn't going to be able to have enough years. Now he sees a whole different possibility. Pretty powerful! So I acknowledge you for being here. This is a courageous journey. This is not for the timid or the weak of heart - just to warn you right now. You are going to be involved in doing some very in-depth stuff - some powerful things that will really make a profound and lasting difference. You'll be challenged. You will! There will be this little monkey...

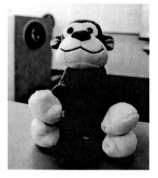

Now, we've all heard of Jiminy Cricket, the little guy who represented a guiding positive consciousness to Pinocchio. Well, we've also got a little monkey, otherwise known as the monkey mind. It sits right here (on your shoulder), and it will say all kinds of things. This little monkey can be rather mischievous and cause all kinds of havoc. "Well, maybe... but I'm not sure about this." "No, that doesn't sound right." "No, I can't possibly do that!" You'll have all of those three sets of conversations going on. We'll just have to deal with the monkey mind. So, I'm going to leave this monkey here to remind you. Anytime you have a conversation going on inside your head and your little monkey is saying, "What are you asking me to do?" Recognizing that it's just the little monkey can help you.

Take a moment and write down right now what you most want to get from being in this program. This may change over time. You may want to get even more. I want you to be aware of what you most want to get out of being in this program starting now.

What I want most by participating in this program is:

_____

_____

In the early 80's, I became an avid follower of Dr. Denis Waitley's methods for studying and producing winning results. Dr. Waitley has his doctorate in Behavioral Psychology, and among many notable accomplishments, was twice the behavioral psychologist for the U.S. Olympic Team. Every athlete that worked with Dr. Waitley attained an Olympic medal. And, all of the U.S. medal winners had worked with Dr. Waitley. He was the master of creating breakthroughs in performance! As a swimming coach of high-level athletes, I learned from Dr. Waitley many facets of empowering athletes to creating breakthroughs in performance. Over the years, I have learned to incorporate many of these "performance breakthrough" insights in working with my athletes, in my work experience and with my clients.

This program is structured into three major parts. The first part is the first three chapters, which are about dealing with what's in between our two ears. We will deal with addressing the mindset, the thinking, and attitudes that will actually make a difference in creating a breakthrough in your health, energy, and vitality. If we don't address this, any action that we take will be on top of that subconscious wiring, and we end up sabotaging ourselves over and over and over again. Are you familiar with that tale? We're going to end that. We're going to really work in-depth.

The first chapter is creating breakthroughs, establishing the foundation for optimal health and vitality. We're going to look at what's at the source of creating a breakthrough and understanding how we sabotage ourselves.

The second chapter will deal with the overall context of the conversation that is pervasive in our culture today. We'll look at the context of scarcity and we'll completely transform that into a conversation for sufficiency – a powerful conversation that we'll have.

The third chapter is really in-depth. You'll get the chance to look at your own personal individual blueprint that you created - not consciously – but that you created nonetheless, based on your experiences of what you heard, what you saw, and what you experienced. As a result of this process, you'll get an opportunity to actually create a new blueprint - a new foundation for creating your life in a whole new powerful way.

You'll be able to create greater health with a whole different level of consciousness.

Then we move into the next seven chapters. These chapters are going to deal with understanding the way our bodies work and the actions and behaviors for greater health. Now, these are all based on solid science. There's no gimmicks, no fads, no blue pills, no magic powder. It's none of that. It's all very solid stuff.

We'll delve into the overall design of the human body in chapter four. The fifth chapter will deal with effective fat reduction for a lifetime. It's called Beyond Dieting. In the sixth chapter we focus on one subject – nutrition - and it's rather extensive. The seventh chapter will be dealing with supplementation. The eight chapter will address the importance of cardiovascular exercise. The ninth chapter will deal with strength and flexibility. In fact, I'm going to teach you how to do a total body workout in just three moves! Can you believe it? It is possible, and it will be amazing! Chapter ten will completely shift how you relate to people and the stress in your life. It's called Powerful Living. It's an amazing chapter.

Then chapter eleven will be spent on creating the new structure - a new framework for sustainability with support, structure and accountability. Because, if you don't have a structure for sustainability with support and accountability, guess what? It's a bold, crazy, wild, amazing idea that you may try that may last a couple weeks. Then what? Then it goes back to the way was before. What we're going to do is create a new structure. And, you're going to be powerfully trained in getting related to your calendar.

I sometimes actually teach CEOs and executives time-management and being able to manage their schedule in a whole different way. We're going to apply it to your health. We're going to actually establish a strategic set of goals for your health. You'll get to do that in chapter eleven. Then you'll have a chance to go and be out in your life and see how it works.

This is not the kind of program where you read, learn, get lots of information, and then I tell you what to do and leave you hanging saying "good luck, good bye, see you later and hope it works out well for you." No! My intention is that we build a community where people learn how to support each other in a sustainable way.

CHAPTER 1

CREATING BREAKTHROUGHS

I'm going to start off with a few questions...

What has been a health challenge or a set of challenges that you've had?

What actions have you taken or avoided taking in regards to this particular challenge that you have been faced with - whatever that challenge is?

Also, how long has it been this way for you?

These challenges have been around for a while, haven't they? They have persisted and they've been consistent over time. You've been working at trying to resolve these problems for quite some time, haven't you? You've been doing a lot of different things or avoiding doing a lot of different things. But, there's been a pattern of actions that you have taken for quite some time, haven't you? And, you haven't gotten any really satisfying results.

Einstein is quoted as saying that *"Insanity is doing the same things over and over again expecting different results."* Now, I'm not going to try to practice Psychiatry here and suggest that you are clinically insane with a DSM-IV diagnosis of a psychiatric disorder. No. But what I will suggest is that we psychologically get conditioned by our patterns of thinking and patterns of behavior such that it becomes the status quo – even though we may not like it. This is the level of insanity that Einstein referred to.

This area that isn't working - we tolerate it. We put up with it. We continue going along the same path and we don't change it. Or we try, but then eventually we give up. If we continue to do what we've always done, then we'll continue to get the same results, over and over again.

In this program, we are out to stop the insanity! Stop it - like no kidding – we're going to stop it! We're really going to examine "What will it take to stop the insanity?" We have to be willing to take a radically different approach.

Einstein said *"The significant problems we face*

cannot be solved at the same level of thinking we were at when we created them." Now examine this quote very carefully. What is Einstein telling us here? To try something different – absolutely. What else is he saying? Ahhh! That we created our own problems! Realize they weren't consciously created, right? Nobody at the age of twenty says "Oh, I think I'm going to have heart disease, diabetes, gain an extra 75 pounds of weight, and I'm going to have a miserable life and have a heart attack by the time I'm 55." Who would create that consciously? None of us, right? But does it happen? You better believe it! We created our own problems. What Einstein was telling us was that we have to recognize that we created our own problems. There was a level of thinking that we were at when we created them. It wasn't conscious. It wasn't intentional. It was all in the subconscious and unconscious level.

We think we are operating at the conscious level all the time. No. What determines who we are right now in the present moment - only 10% is from our conscious mind, 60% of what's running us is from our subconscious mind, and 30% is from our unconscious mind. Interesting, isn't it? 90% of what's running you in any given moment - you don't even know it's running you. Pretty amazing isn't it? We have to get that the significant problems we face require a different level of thinking and accepting the responsibility for the fact that we created the problem, because there was a particular level of thinking we were at when we created them. It wasn't intentional, but we created it nonetheless. If we accept that fact, then we have power in the matter. We now are empowered to do something about it. Instead of trying to blame the government, or McDonald's, or whoever - instead of blaming anything else, we can take responsibility.

The purpose for this chapter is to 1) empower you in shifting your thinking so that you can actually create a breakthrough in your health, energy and vitality, 2) to establish a foundation for understanding how we sabotage ourselves, and 3) the key pillars for success.

Now, let's talk about what it takes to create a breakthrough and how to access this.

Defining breakthrough

Let's begin by defining a breakthrough. A breakthrough can mean lots of things – an 'aha' moment, a profound shift, a paradigm shift and other possible definitions. All of these are valid interpretations of what a breakthrough means. But, for the purposes of this conversation, let's use the metaphor of breaking through a board as in a martial arts demonstration. I'm sure you've seen that before.

Let's just say that I am holding a typical wooden board out in front of you. It's about 12 inches by 12 inches and about an inch thick. I'm going to brace myself and hold the board up for you to break with your hand. But first, I need to ask, what will be your point of focus? Where will you be focusing your attention?

If you have never broken a board before and you're like most people, you would likely focus your attention on the center of the board. That's the most common response. However, that's what will prevent you from breaking the board.

What most of us do in life is the same thing. We focus on the barriers or problems represented by the board. We put our time and attention on the problem. We put our energy on the problem. We put our resources on the problem. And, we end up with more of... you guessed it – more of the problem! We just never get past the problem.

The secret to breaking the board is to focus our attention where? beyond the board – beyond the problem. The paradox here is that you need to know where the board is in order to focus past it. Likewise, you need to focus past the problem in order to get past the problem. Therefore, in order to achieve a breakthrough we need to focus at a whole different level than what we may be accustomed to.

We can now define a breakthrough as **breaking through a resistance or a barrier giving us access to a new dimension or a new arena that was previously unseen or undiscovered**. It gives us access to a new dimension – a whole different arena.

Einstein said that *"Imagination is more important than knowledge. For knowledge is limited, whereas imagination embraces the entire world, stimulating progress, giving birth to evolution."*

Imagination is what leads to creativity and innovation which is where real progress is made. Yet, we tend to seek out more information and knowledge in an attempt to break through the "board."

For instance, we have more information, more books, more infomercials, more programs, more exercises, more pills than ever before to address weight loss. Yet, obesity and being overweight continues to rise in the United States. Clearly, more knowledge does not make a difference!

What we need to recognize is that knowledge is inherently limited – there is only so much we can acquire. Therefore, we have to tap into the domain of imagination, creativity and innovation in order to evolve into a whole new level of success. But since we can't seem to do this on our own, how do we gain access to this domain?

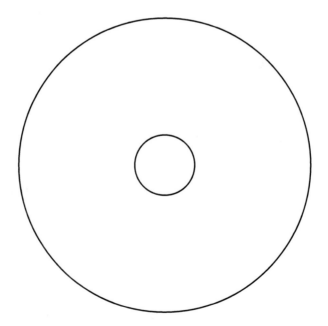

Domain of imagination, creativity and innovation

My physics teacher at St. John Bosco High School, Brother Gene Mylan, who had his Ph.D. in physics from Notre Dame University and was a Carnegie Institute researcher, drew this diagram for us in class one day.

The inner circle represents what we know, and you'll notice that it's fairly small, for our knowledge is limited. The outer circle contains what we don't know and we're generally aware of this. This area is limited as well. What Einstein was referring to was the area outside of these circles, which extends with no limits beyond the outer circle. This is the area of imagination that "embraces the entire world, stimulating progress, giving birth to evolution." This is the area for us to tap into in order for us to continually evolve.

But, how do we do that? Psychological research shows that most of us as adults have lost this innate sense of imagination, creativity and innovation that we once had as little children. As adults, this domain of imagination is generally hidden to us, and we are blind to it.

Johari Window

For this, we'll look at something frequently used in management training called the Johari Window.

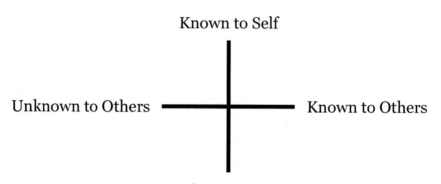

What is known to ourselves and known to others - we know it, they know it - this is public information. Everybody knows it. What's known to ourselves but unknown to others - we know it, they don't -therefore it's private. What's unknown to ourselves and unknown to others at this point, is unknowable. It's the area of discovery. But the area of interest is the area that is known to others yet is unknown to ourselves. We don't know it, but others do. This is the area of our blind spot. This is what gives us access to breakthroughs. It's being able to access what others can see that we can't see for ourselves. It's driving behind the car that is about to change lanes into somebody else's space; they're trying to change lanes into a blind spot. It gives us access, and we have to be able to get access to something that somebody else can see that we can't.

Now, I've got this little exercise. I have a single nail being balanced on the head of this nail.

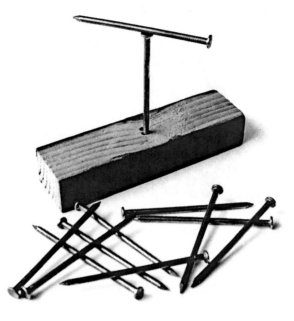

However, it is possible to balance all eleven of these nails simultaneously on the head of that nail. Do you know how to do it? Either you know it or you don't. It is possible to do it. This is in the domain of what is known to others but it unknown to yourself. Using the principles of engineering, of balance and counter-balance, it is possible to balance all of these nails simultaneously on the head of this nail. Now my uncle was a professor of civil engineering at the University of Texas in Houston and he built bridges and roads. If you drive over the Golden Gate Bridge or the Bay Bridge, you will notice that the same principles are being utilized in those bridges (suspension bridges).

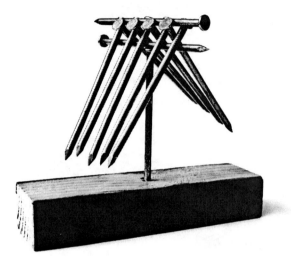

Now you can see that all of these nails are balanced on the head of that single nail. This is how it's done. This is an example of something that you didn't know, isn't it?

So what gives us access to a breakthrough, is what's available to others that they can see but you can't see for yourself. Simply put, it's not going to be in the domain of knowing, okay? Because there is only so much knowledge that you can cram into your cranium, right? Only so much. You can only study so much. I learned that one in medical school – there was only so much information we could take on. That was it. It was impossible to take it all on. And, it's not in the actions either. Interestingly enough, a lot of times we hear someone tell us, "oh, you just have to do this or you just have to do that", and you try it for a couple weeks and it goes right back to the way it was before. So you'll get short term results at best. So it's not in the actions either. What has to shift is the thinking, that's first.

Therefore, **what empowers us to produce a breakthrough is a willingness to be receptive to what others can see that we can't see for ourselves**. As my great mentor, former UCLA Coach John Wooden said, "It is what you learn after you know it all that counts." This is what Coach Wooden defined as "being willing to be coachable."

I coached swimming for nearly 30 years. I've been a high level coach - a fanatic if you will. In fact I was so fanatical that I wrote two books on the subject of stroke technique. The first one was in 1998. The second edition is called The Swimming Drill Book. It's the only comprehensive drill book for competitive swimming in the world. It's been translated to Italian, Japanese, Portuguese, and soon to be in Spanish. Well over 55,000 copies sold already for a training book - that's pretty darn good.

Being coachable

What gives us access to a breakthrough in performance of any kind, is being willing to be coachable. I remember when Summer Sanders was only thirteen years old. Now if you know swimming, you know that Olympic gold medalist, Summer Sanders, came out of the Roseville area. She swam right here in Sacramento. In 1992 she was a two-time gold medalist. Now, at thirteen, did she know everything there was to know about being an Olympic gold medalist? Don't think so. But she became one. What gave her access? Being coachable. I happen to know her coaches, and she was extremely coachable. Mike Hastings and Richard Quick were her coaches. Phenomenal athlete. Therefore, what gives us access to breakthroughs is really being willing to be coachable. That's what's really important. We have to be willing.

What I've discovered over the years of coaching athletes and high performance people, is that there are four distinct levels of coachability.

The first level of coachability is, simply, **not coachable**. Now you probably know people like this. They are uncoachable because they listen to one voice only – their own. Their own little voice, that's it, they don't listen to anyone else. Right? So they listen to their own little voice, they're not listening to anybody. They're not coachable.

The second level of coachability is what's called **selectively coachable**. Selectively coachable means that they'll listen to the coach, and do what the coach asks them to do, when they agree with it. The rest of the time, who are they listening to? Their own little voice. That's how it works. By the way, how many of you are employers? You know this is what you have to deal with, isn't it? As a leader, a business owner, business entrepreneur, you have to deal with people knowing that their own little voice is who they're going to listen to most of the time. By the way, as human beings, this is how we operate.

We're either not coachable, or selectively coachable, at best, by default. That's how we are wired.

It takes courage to step into the third level. The third level of coachability is **reluctantly coachable**. Reluctantly coachable means that you'll do everything the coach asks you to do, whether you like it or not. You'll do it willingly. You still have a little voice that's saying things like, "I don't know if this is going to work", "I don't know if I can do this", "I don't know if I'm good enough", "I don't know if this person really knows what they're talking about", "I'll try it for six weeks and if it doesn't work, I'll go back to my old ways". So there's the voice of doubt. And it happens to be there when we're reluctantly coachable.

The quantum shift occurs in becoming **completely coachable**. That's an extremely rare level. Completely coachable means that you actually do everything the coach asks you to do. You actually empower your coach to win. Because when your coach wins, then you win too. You take the focus off of you and your little voice. You surrender the little voice.

Which level of coachability do you think it takes to actually reach the Olympic games? Completely coachable – nothing less. Have you watched the Winter or Summer Olympics? It's amazing, right? These are amazing athletes. The snowboarding alone – they're going off a half pipe and flying through the air – holy Toledo! I know how to ski, but I'm not going there. It's amazing what some of these people can do. Amazing. The ice skating, the luge – traveling at 100 miles per hour on the ice? Are you kidding? It's incredible. It takes being completely coachable to get to that level, and nothing short of that.

I was very fortunate growing up. My father was the undefeated, two year, welterweight, Golden Gloves boxing champion in Mexico. By the way, they take their boxing very seriously in Mexico. And he was an alternate for the Olympic games. He came to this country when he was only 19. Because he was such an amazing athlete, he got the chance to learn how to play tennis from a man by the name of Poncho Segura. If you know tennis, you know that Poncho Segura was a five-time Wimbledon champion and trained more Wimbledon champions than any other coach, even to this day. He coached Jimmy Connors, he coached Poncho Gonzalez, and a whole bunch of other people. Here I am, I'm five years old, I'm going with my father to watch him play tennis, and I'm throwing tennis balls to the likes of Stan Smith, Billie Jean King, Rod Laver; I didn't know who they were! But I got to be around them. Do you think that was a different environment? Yes, pretty extraordinary.

Becoming completely coachable is not something that you can flip a switch and "there it is." It's not something where you walk in and say, "Ruben, work with me, I'm completely coachable". Nice try. It's not that easy. It is a process and it takes a lot of hard work. There's growth in the process, and there has to be a committed coach in the process as well.

Jon's story

In 1993, I had a young man come and work for me as an assistant coach, his name was Jon Piland. Now, when I first met Jon he wasn't that impressive. He rolled up on his motorcycle, long blonde hair streaming out of his helmet, he'd just finished cleaning a swimming pool. He had a resume that was folded and wrinkled and handed it to me. This was a private club. I opened up the resume and I noticed something. Three years earlier, he had been a member of the national record-setting 200 meter medley relay team. And he was the breaststroker. No small feat. I got to working with him - he was great with the kids. Then I said, "Jon, you're in great shape. I have to watch you swim. Just humor me, okay?" So, I watched him swim. Now, have you ever seen the potential that somebody has? You see it, but they can't see it for themselves? You see it in the moment. Have you had that experience? Amazing, isn't it? It took me all of thirty seconds. He got done and the first thing I did was think "Thank you, God!", because as a coach I typically worked for years in developing talent. It's nice to get it in your lap once in a while. It really is. I got him out of the water and I said, "Look, you're not done yet. You're 21 years old. You're in your prime. You've got the body of a god, all right. You can do anything if you put your mind to it. But I'm clear you lost your dream along the way. What was your dream?" And what he shared with me was that his dream was to reach the Olympic trials. He knew he had it in him to get to the Olympic trials. I said, "Look, you have three years. You can do it. But it's going to take three things. ***Number one, you're going to have to learn a whole new, different set of skills. That, I can teach you. Secondly, you're going to need to be willing to work harder than you've ever worked in your life. There is no substitute for industriousness and hard work. Thirdly, you're going to need to be willing to be coachable.*** Now, it's just a willingness to be coachable. I don't expect people to be completely coachable right off the bat. That's asking too much. But a willingness to be coachable, just being willing." Jon said yes, that he would agree to that, and I said yes, too. Then we created a sacred pact. It was sort of like the karate kid, the bandana and the sponge - it was sort of like that.

The only time that summer we could get into the pool was at 5:30 in the morning. We had an hour and a half from 5:30 until 7:00 – that was it. 5:30 in the morning! Do you know what 5:30 in the morning in a swimming pool feels like? Now here's the thing. I knew that he had three years of experience of being not coachable, so I knew he was going to be selectively coachable at best. There were some mornings I was there at 5:30 in the morning; where do you think Jon was? He was still in bed. What do you think I was doing at 5:35? That's right – calling him.

"Jon, get your butt out of bed, get down here!" Good thing he only lived a couple blocks away. Point is, I had to hold him accountable to his dream. You get what I'm saying here? Because without that accountability and support, guess where

Jon would be today? Someplace else.

Audience: You were more committed than he was.

Exactly. And I told him that several times. He didn't understand it at the time – I was more committed to him than he was to himself. I had to be. I had to hold the space for his dream. In fact there were a couple times where he'd just disappear for a whole week, and I'd welcome him back. He was the like the prodigal son, I'd welcome him back every single time. Because, I knew this was going to happen. I could expect it, he's a human being.

After about a year, Jon stepped into being reluctantly coachable - the next stage. He started doing everything he needed to do. Everything. All the workouts, all the diet, all the strength training, all the flexibility. He started doing everything. But he still had the voice of doubt. "I don't know if I can do it. I don't know if I'm going to be able to make it. I don't know if this is going to work. I have such a long way to go." And he said those things all the time. It was all good. We had lots of conversations about it. And, I supported him.

Then, in 1995, he stepped into being completely coachable. It was awesome. It was a quantum shift. It was just an amazing shift. He made Nationals both times that year. And, in the spring of 1996, Jon Piland was the final person to qualify for the US Olympic trials by four-hundredths of a second. Not a whole lot of time folks. But he made it. He was there. And when he actually swam in Indianapolis he was acknowledged with a standing ovation because no one, that we knew of, had quit the sport for three years, trained for three years, and made it to the Olympic trials.

Surviving vs. Thriving

"All of life is in one of two states. Either it is surviving or it is thriving, and that's all there is." – Dr. Michael Kolitsky, my professor of Biological Sciences and mentor at California Lutheran University. I suggest that being completely coachable gives us access to a whole different level of thinking and believing in oneself that I call Thriving. But in order to understand Thriving, we need to contrast it to Surviving.

Psychological research shows that most of us, most of the time are surviving – living in fear. Medical research shows that chronic disease is really caused by being chronically stressed and in survival. Our bodies are at dis-ease! What this looks like is that we become attached to our wants, desires, judgments, assessments, worries, concerns, complaints, issues, cynicism, skepticism, criticism, resignation, blame, shame, guilt, etc, etc. Get the picture? It's just such a limiting state of mind. And, it's rather common. It's what you get when you turn on the television. It's what you get on all the talk shows. It's what you get in the newspaper. It's what you get in the magazines. It's just all around us.

The other possible mindset is that of Thriving. In this mindset, we live what Stephen Covey calls a "principle-centered life," based on principles such as integrity, honesty, trust, responsibility, generosity, kindness, and compassion. How it looks is that we actually live our lives by honoring our promises, commitments and agreements. I remember that my father used to say "a man is only as good as his word." He was a champion, and this is how champions think and act. I happen to know a few Olympians, and this is how they think and act also. And, I've coached and developed many champions over the years. This is an uncommon way of thinking, yet anyone can take this on. Anyone!

I got the chance to meet Jose Hernandez in 2010. From a migrant farm working family, grew up in Stockton, but because of the extraordinary way that his parents viewed him and how they trained him to view himself, he ended up becoming an astronaut for NASA and had a mission in 2008 on the space station. How is it that a poor child, born in Mexico, to migrant farm workers, ends up in the space station for NASA? Is it from the mindset of survival? I don't think so. It's from the mindset of thriving.

Arms exercise

We're going to do a little exercise. Here's what we're going to do. Everybody stand up. This exercise actually comes from an Olympian. Stand up, make sure you're standing nice, straight and tall. You're going to need to have a little wingspan so make sure you don't hit somebody. Lift your arms up now to shoulder height. Take your right index finger and touch the tip of your nose. And back out. Left index finger, touch the tip of your nose, and back out. Very good, you're all sober, I'm glad to see that. Now, research shows that if you can do those actions, you can hold your arms up at shoulder height for at least two minutes.

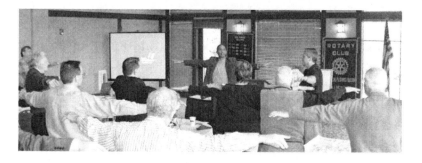

Now, notice where your little voice went. There're two choices that you have. One is the voice of defeat which lives in the realm of survival and says, "Two minutes, are you crazy? No way I'm going to be able to do this." That's the voice of survival. The other option is the voice of thriving, or the voice of victory that says, "Okay, two minutes, I'm all right, bring it on. If Roger's doing it, I'm going to do it." So turn and face a partner. And have a conversation. Now here's the question: What would be possible if you could actually operate from the state of thriving all the time? What kind of difference could that make in your health, your energy and your vitality? Are you ready? Go!

Tic, toc, tic, toc....

Put your arms down, have a quick seat for a second. By the way, you went for two minutes and fifteen seconds. I just want to hear from a few of you. What would be possible if you could operate from the mindset of thriving? What kinds of things would be possible?

Audience members:

> "Changing your life!"
> "Be more positive!"
> "I wouldn't be so stressed!"
> "Absolutely anything that I want!"

Yes! Absolutely anything that you want would be possible. And anything in relation to your health, your energy, your vitality would be possible. Write down what you can now see would be possible for your health, energy and vitality. Capture this moment, now!

3 Elements of a breakthrough

When we look now at creating a breakthrough, we can see from this conversation that there are three elements that are necessary to create a breakthrough.

Number one, there has to be a shift in mind set, attitude and thinking. That has to happen in between our ears. That has to happen first. Second, we have to have a corresponding shift in actions and behaviors. It has to correspond. It has to match up. We can't think one way and act differently, that's not going to work. It has to be corresponding. Now, many bright people are usually capable of accomplishing the first two steps, but it doesn't seem to stick. That's because there's another piece. Third, we've got to create a new structure for support and accountability. Without the support and accountability the shifts in mindset and behaviors wither to oblivion. They do not come into full fruition. We have to be able to sustain those new practices. That's what is required.

The Mechanism of Self-Sabotage

The crux of the matter, however, is this – whether we know what to do or not, we still manage to sabotage ourselves. This is a subconscious process. It's because there are some persistent conversations that we have with ourselves. That little voice that says the same things at certain times, especially in the moment of truth. "Do I go to the gym or do I go to Baskin-Robbins? Maybe I should do both? Maybe I'll go to Baskin-Robbins first." These are the conversations that we all have.

Go back to the challenge that we talked about in the beginning. In the moment of truth, when you're in that state of survival, when you are challenged by whatever it is that your challenge is, the one that's been there for quite some time, what is it that you are saying to yourself? This is a subconscious conversation. It's your little monkey's voice. By the way, this is not pretty.

Audience members: "I think my body will go into shock if

I stopped doing everything bad and started doing everything good to it.

      It won't matter.

      Just for now.

      I deserve it.

      I'll start tomorrow.

      I'll work out more later.

      I need it.

      I'm tired of denying myself.

      Everyone else is doing it."

Can you relate to these? It's what we all do. Our little voice goes off. The little monkey is loose and very mischievous. In the moment of truth we have all these kinds of conversations with ourselves. It's a common process. It's how we all are as human beings. These conversations are fairly persistent – they appear over and over again. We continue to hold on to these conversations. There's a reason for this.

Consider for a moment that how we operate as human beings, even at the subconscious level, there's always "what's in it for me?" There's something that we're getting out of holding on to these conversations. There is some payoff. And it could be a whole list of payoffs. This is all a subconscious process – you would not consciously do this. If you did, you would've had it handled by now. There is a group of subconscious payoffs that your little monkey gets, and this is the nasty side of how we are as human beings. It's just how we're wired.

Here are some of the **most common subconscious payoffs**:

- Instant gratification, I want it and I want it now, I deserve it now.

- Comfort, ease and laziness. We get to be comfortable. We get to be lazy; we get to have it our way.

- We get to justify ourselves, we have our reasons that we feel are perfectly valid. And we invalidate anyone who says otherwise. "I deserve to have that Pepsi Cola with the double cheeseburger. I deserve it."

- When we have our reasons, we hold on to our reasons for dear life, therefore, we get to be right. By the way, we go to war just to be right. People die just to be right. It's amazing what we do just to be right.

- If we are in that competitive mindset, it's all about winning. We have to win and be superior.

- If we do that, it's all about being in control. We delude ourselves so we think we're in control. It's a delusion, and ultimately it's about avoiding responsibility. We get to shirk responsibility for ourselves. "No, you made me the way that I am, it's not me." Therefore, we avoid responsibility and become inferior.

- As Colin Tipping, author of *Radical Forgiveness, Radical Manifestation*, and a few other books, wrote that the ultimate payoffs are that we get to perpetuate being a victim, a martyr or a rescuer. "I'm suffering because of my circumstances – woe is me!" Or we say,

"There's so much that I have to take care of, all these people, my children, my family, everything else. I can't possibly take care of me. There is no time for me." And so we play the martyr. The other is being the rescuer, thinking "I can save them" even to our own detriment. These are very common roles, and we adopt them as human beings.

Which of these payoffs is your little monkey getting fed by? Make a note. There's usually a pattern.

Now, what keeps these payoffs in place are **three primary subconscious conversations**.

1. "I'm not getting what I want." The little monkey is like a three year old and there is somebody or something getting in the way of what you want. Some desire is blocked.

2. "It shouldn't be this way." The little monkey gets attached to an expectation of how life should be. "You should do this, you should do that, they should do this, they shouldn't do that..." Basically, the little monkey "shoulds" all over you! Yet, who among us is qualified to determine how life should be for anyone else? No one! Yet, I'm sure you know plenty of people who operate as if their opinion is the supreme opinion on the planet!

3. "Don't say anything. It will only make it worse. It won't matter. Why bother?" The little monkey stuffs and suppresses communication as a defense mechanism. It often will hold back from communication until a certain

incident will cause a volcanic eruption or until there is just a choking of communication. "Withholding and supressing is to relationships like rat poison is to rats. It leads to a slow, certain and painful death!" - Coach Ruben

Make note of which of these conversations you recognize for yourself. Again, there is usually a pattern.

What's at the foundation of it all is FEAR. Fear keeps us in survival and using this mechanism of self-sabotage. There are five major fears that stop us and keep us from realizing our goals.

1. Fear of failure
2. Fear of rejection
3. Fear of success
4. Fear of the unknown
5. Fear of being uncomfortable

Make note of which of these fears you recognize for yourself. Again, there is usually a pattern.

Now, when your subconscious, your monkey mind, is operating and getting these payoffs, it's costing you. There's a toll, a detriment, an impact. You're losing out. What are you losing out on? In the moment of truth, when you're holding on to these payoffs, you're holding on to these conversations, you're holding on to these fears, what are you losing out on?

Good health, vitality, confidence, peace, energy, time, money, aliveness, productivity, happiness, activity, community, and lots more.

Write down what you can see for yourself that are some of the things it's costing you. What's it costing you when you hold on to that little voice and the payoffs you're getting?

Nearly 30 years ago, a very dear teacher of mine, Jim Rohn said, that *"for everything in life, we have one of two price tags to pay. It's either the pain of regret or the joy from discipline. That's it. And if you don't like it, you have to move to a different planet."* Many of us don't know what the joy from discipline is even like because we get so caught up in the instant gratification and being comfortable and being lazy, etc. We get used to that. We get trained in that. But there is a particular joy that emerges from discipline. It emerges from the consistent practice of being in the state of thriving. It's a whole different level.

My swimmers used to come to practice and they'd ask, "Coach, can we have fun today?" And I'd say, "Your form of fun or my form of fun?" I trained them hard because I wanted them to experience the joy from discipline. The joy that comes from being committed to excellence and leads to achieving such tremendous levels of accomplishment. I'd say. "I'm training you to have an experience of joy and fun that you don't even know is available to you yet. If you work really, really hard, you'll get to qualify to go to the National Age Group Championships. We'll get to go on that trip to Monterey, we'll get to go on that trip to Phoenix, Arizona. We'll get to go on that trip to Nationals and you'll get to experience meeting people from all over the world. But if we have your kind of fun today and it's a cheap, easy fun and we don't train hard, we'll never get to those wondrous places and experience that amazing level that most people only dream of."

You get to choose. From this moment onward you're going to start to hear your little monkey a little more often. This is kind of the curse of this program. You're going to hear your little monkey and in that moment, you're going to recognize it. A Buddhist principle is that awareness is the first step towards enlightenment. When you become aware of your little monkey, you're empowered to start taking a different course of action. Awareness is the key, and you'll get to choose which path you want to go on. And the choice is always yours. There's only one thing you have to do after your born. What is it? Die. They put you in a hole, they throw dirt on your face and they have a party anyways. Everything in between is your choice. It's always your choice. *Whether you think you have a choice or not, the reality is you always have a choice.* You hear people say, "Well I had no choice in the matter." That is a bunch of hooey. Not true. You always have a choice. You may not like the consequences, you may not prefer those consequences, but you always have a choice.

What will it take for you to be successful?

The first pillar of success is **integrity**. This is key. Stephen Covey, who wrote the Seven Habits of Highly Successful People, said that the ability to make promises to oneself and keep them is the foundation of living an extraordinary life. It's being true to your word. You make a promise to yourself and you keep it. It's the hardest thing to do because as human beings we sabotage ourselves, we lie to ourselves all the time. It's not bad, it's just human.

The second pillar is **commitment**. Commitment is about dedication to the long term course of action. It's about action, not a resolution. It's not a wish. It's not a statement or a goal – it's about being in action. It's about starting exercise tomorrow; you put it in your planner and you actually schedule it. You get into action and you actually do it. That's commitment. Otherwise it's just a goal on a piece of paper. "Someday I'll exercise." It doesn't carry any weight. Never, ever, ever, ever, ever give up. Never give up. If you think you're not doing well, still, never give up.

The third pillar is **being coachable**. Being coachable means finding the best coach available (of course that would be me!) and completely trusting your coach. And you should probably empower yourself with many coaches. I have several, yes, even I have coaches. I am coachable. I could not be a good coach if I was not coachable myself. You need to embrace many coaches, wherever you possibly can. It's important to do that. Trust your coach, empower your coach to win, then you win too. Take the attention off of you in doing what the coach asks you to do. You'll be amazed at your results when you do it that way.

There's an old Buddhist saying, "To know and not to use is to not yet to know". Your homework is not about reading this book and just getting information. The program lives in your life when you're not reading this book. That is the program. This time that you're reading is the huddle. The playing field is out there in your life. We come together here when you're reading. You regroup, you get centered, you figure out your strategy and you go out there and get on the field and get going.

Your mission, should you choose to accept it:

1. Practice giving up your excuses, justifications and complaints. Another teacher of mine is Edwene Gaines. She wrote The Four Spiritual Laws of Prosperity, fabulous book. Amazing. Here's the challenge. Take on being complaint free for thirty days in a row. You make so much as one complaint on day 29, you start over. Thirty days in a row. I promise it will completely alter your life. When you're in complaint mode, you're in the domain of the ordinary. You're in survival.

2. Second, practice choosing the joy of discipline. When you're in that moment of truth and you hear that little voice, you get to choose. Make the tough choice. Choose discipline, not regret. And sometimes it's a more difficult choice. Be willing to take that on for yourself.

3. Third, practice thriving. Live life based on principles, and be "as good as your word." This is a tall order. It's a practice.

Notice I say practice. There's no expectation to be perfect at all, that's not the program. The program is about being in practice. The swimmer that comes into a competitive program at eight years of age is not going to be an Olympian in two years. There's a lot more practice that needs to happen before that's even going to possibly occur. This whole program is about being in practice.

We'll finish this chapter with a quote from Murray on commitment:

"Until one is committed, there is hesitancy, the chance to draw back. Concerning all acts of initiative and creation, there is one elementary truth, that ignorance of which kills countless ideas and splendid plans. That the moment one definitely commits oneself, then providence moves too. All sorts of things occur to help one that would never otherwise have occurred. A whole stream of events, issues from the decision raising in one's favor all manner of unforeseen incidents and meetings and material assistance which no one could have dreamt would have come their way. Whatever you can do, or dream you can do, begin it. Boldness has genius, power, and magic in it. Begin it now."

CHAPTER 2

THE SOUL OF FITNESS

In this chapter, we're going to work at creating a new context for health and fitness. First, we'll be looking at the cultural context or the cultural conversation that is pervasive in our entire Western culture that really is at the source of what holds us back. Then we'll create a new context. In the next chapter we're going to take a look at the individual blueprint that we each have individually created, and that's called the Secrets of the Fit Mind.

We'll start off with some questions that you should ask yourself.

When things are not going well in regards to your health, what do you say to yourself? What is that little monkey's voice saying at those moments?

"I'll never be able to get enough time to exercise." "It's just too hard to eat healthy." Whatever the case may be, what are those conversations that you have with yourself? Take a moment to write these down.

The usual process for how we address the problems that we're faced with is to usually just talk about it first. We talk about our problems to other people. We share our problems because God knows that misery loves company. Then we sometimes try to do more. We'll take some actions seeing if we can resolve our problems and our issues in order to have more success. However, we generally do not address the mindset. We seldom change the mindset. We try to do more and we talk about it more, but we don't really do what we need to actually make a change.

Mindset

Let's consider for a moment that the mindset is what needs to be shifted here. As Bob Proctor of *The Secret* says, we need to establish a new paradigm – a new way of thinking. A new framework for how we think.

Think about a room – any bedroom in your house. Let's say that the bedroom is filled with certain pieces of furniture – a bed, a dresser, a chair and a night stand. Now, it's possible for us to rearrange the furniture in the room, but the walls of the room still remain the same. The walls define the limits of the room. The walls are the framework. Therefore, the walls determine what you can do with the room. We can call the walls the context and the furniture the content. The context determines the limits of what you can do with the content.

Your mindset is like the walls in a room. This mental framework or paradigm determines how we view things. From studies in psychology, our thoughts, feelings and actions are usually consistent with our mindset. Otherwise, it leads to what is called "cognitive dissonance," and we struggle to resolve the inconsistencies between our beliefs and actions.

Lynn Twist, who wrote a book called *The Soul of Money*, traveled the world and revealed that there are just two major paradigms around money, but this concept applies to just about anything.

Scarcity

There is a pervasive context in our culture. This context is the context of Scarcity. Scarcity is a conversation that has us, we're actually trapped by this context. We don't see it, we don't see how prevalent it is, but it's all around us in our lives and it's completely pervasive. It's as if we are the fish in a bowl of muddy water – we can't tell that it's muddy, we are just swimming in it and think it's just fine.

Scarcity is kept in place by three myths. **The first myth is that "there's not enough."** We view the world as deficient. We do not have enough. When we're in that place of viewing the world as deficient, it generates a sense of fear, and a sense of survival. We're in survival mode all the time, so it doesn't work for us. Consider the fact that there are many times when we say, "there's not enough". There's not enough time, there's not enough resources, there's not enough gyms, there's not enough whatever. Where do you say that there's not enough of anything? And particularly, where do you say there's not enough in relationship to your health and your fitness? There's not enough good, organic food around, there's not enough recipes, there's not enough good information; whatever the case may be. Make a list of where you say "there's not enough."

The second myth that perpetuates scarcity is the flip side of the coin. On one side we have 'there's not enough', the flip side is **"I need more, I want more, I should have more."** On one side there's not enough, and the converse is that we need more. We need more of the same things we've been thinking about. In "I need more, I want more, I should have more." we judge ourselves and compare ourselves to others. It becomes a race with no winners, where we never arrive. We just continue to be like a dog chasing its tail, and that's what we continue to do. Make a list for yourself where you say, "I need more. I want more. I should have more. I need to have more of this."

The third myth that perpetuates scarcity is that **"this is just the way that it is and there's no way out. There's nothing I can do to change it. I give up."** It becomes a place where we start to justify the situation and we start to let go, surrender and give up. It's a place of resignation and hopelessness. We give up trying to change the circumstances, trying to change our lives. You get to the point where you say, "Well, the doctor told me I would never be able to lose weight so I'm just going to give up. I'm not going to worry about it anymore. I'm just going to be overweight." "The doctor told me I would have to be on blood pressure medication for the rest of my life so I'm just giving up. I'm not going to try to empower myself, I'm just giving up." "The doctor told me I'm always going to have back pain, so I'm just giving up. I'm just going to have to live with it." Where have you said "I give up, I surrender?" Where have you become resigned and begun to have a sense of hopelessness about anything, especially in relationship to your health and fitness? Make a list of these.

When we start to look, we can see that we have this whole series of conversations around scarcity. It's really common. We all do this, especially in this culture.

Why does scarcity persist? Why is it maintained for us? It persists because it's all about survival. We get into survival mode and we stay there – we persist being in survival. Life becomes about making it. We're in survival mode, we're in crisis mode, and then we share with our friends and family members and people in our social circles. And, guess what? They're in the same boat as well. There's a lot of agreement. We get plenty of support for us being in scarcity because they're in scarcity, you're in scarcity – the whole world is in scarcity. It's so pervasive and all around us. It's in the newspapers, it's on talk shows, it's on television, it's in just about everything you can think about.

This agreement for scarcity becomes so powerful that we begin to view it as being the truth. It lives for us like it's the truth and yet, it really isn't. It's not the truth at all. Once we see this, once we see that scarcity is just a mythology, it's just a perspective that we've created and bought into. Then we can actually create a new context -. a new direction that we can embrace.

Sufficiency

We've talked about scarcity, we've talked about how pervasive that is. That's the wall. That's the barrier that's in front of us that we hit our head against time and time again. Just like what it takes to break a board, you first need to know where the board is. Now we can see the "board" of scarcity. To break the board, we'll need to focus on a point beyond the board – the point of a new mindset, a new paradigm. What Lynn Twist actually discovered by traveling the world is that there are actually populations of people that live with a different mindset. Their mindset is that there is enough. They don't have this thinking of lack or limitation in their lives at all. They exist as a cohesive group of people living together and working together and it's fascinating to see. There are groups of people that actually live this way.

What she discovered is that there is a possible way of thinking, a way of actually living, called Sufficiency. There is enough of everything that we need, even though resources may be limited (there's only so much of anything), but there is always enough. Many indigenous cultures as well as Native Americans have been living this way forever. They live off the land, there's plenty, there's enough, they use everything and they use it well. We have so much to learn from other cultures.

3 truths of sufficiency

The first truth is that time, money and energy – and everything really is energy - and it's like water. **There is a flow to everything, for everything is always changing.** Nothing is static even though it may appear that way due to our limited senses. For instance, if you set a pen on a table, it may appear like it's not changing. Yet, scientists have calculated that the pen is changing approximately three TRILLION times a second!! At a micro level, every electron in every atom is moving. At a macro level, the location of the pen on the face of the planet is moving at an enormous rate of speed through space.

Everything is energy and there is a flow. It's possible to have either a trickle or a raging current. Did you know that you have a system in your body to create the flow of energy? At the level of your cells – you have a nucleus with genetic material inside, and then you have these little organelles called mitochondria. Mitochondria work if we have oxygen present. We take in our food, break it down and convert it into a human fuel, and then convert this fuel into energy. We take what's called pyruvate, which is the breakdown of glycogen, and we convert it to adenosine triphosphate (ATP), which is the energy molecule in your body. As human beings, we actually run on ATP. Here's the amazing thing. The number of cells in your body stays relatively constant. Or it should once you reach an adult state. If you have a proliferation of cells, we'd call it a cancer or a tumor – you don't want that. The cell number stays constant but the physiology inside the cells can actually be altered. There's a law of the planet – if you don't use, you lose it. The converse of that is that if you do use it, you gain. For example, you cannot increase muscle strength unless you challenge your muscles. The body is designed so that if you use it, you gain. We've taken people who are sedentary and did a muscle biopsy, put it under a microscope and found very few mitochondria per cell – let's say four for this example. Then, we put those people on a cardiovascular exercise program for six months – 5 to 6 days per week, consistently 20 minutes per day – then repeated the muscle biopsy. The mitochondria in the cells had greatly increased – let's say twelve. The analogy is that they went from a 4 cylinder Honda to a 12 cylinder Lamborghini. Which engine uses more fuel even in idle? Which engine is producing more energy? The Lamborghini!

You have an energy system that is meant to be used. This is your design. If you use your design as you were meant to be using it, you actually have the power to increase the flow of energy substantially. It's incredible. And it doesn't cost you anything. No pills, no pharmaceutical drugs, but you will have to put in some sweat and time. We have the capacity to increase the flow of energy within our bodies. Everything in life and nature that we know works on the same principle. *The greater the flow, the greater the power. The question that we have to ask ourselves constantly is "What activities increase the flow?"* One is exercise, another is proper nutrition. Would you believe strength work also contributes? When you put all three together it's a multiplication effect. When you have a balance of everything, the multiplication effect is amazing. You need to do it all.

The second truth of sufficiency is that **what we appreciate, appreciates. This is the law of gratitude. That for which we are grateful for actually expands in kind**. In fact, that which we put our attention to grows in same direction as our attention. Whatever we put our positive time, money, energy and attention to, flourishes. The more we appreciate, the greater the value. So many of us get caught up in the scarcity context and we don't love ourselves. We start being critical of our bodies. We start being critical of what we don't have, instead of appreciating what we do have. We need to be grateful for what we do have. When we start to go down this path, it's amazing what starts to shift. We need to practice what we're grateful for.

If you don't know my car, you'd know it because it has four bumper stickers on it – "If not for love, then why?" "Anything is possible." "What are you grateful for?" and "Go vegan." There's a wonderful little prayer that I say to myself every day. I learned it awhile back and it's really been powerful for me

41

in my life. I say, *"Thank you, God, for everything. My life is completely wonderful, I have no complaints whatsoever."* It's powerful to get grounded in loving everything and everybody because then you can love yourself that much more.

The third truth is that **collaboration creates prosperity**. When we're caught up in scarcity, we're in a silo. We're in a little place and we're trying to do it all by ourselves. We're thinking, "woe is me, no one loves me, I'll never be able to do this." We don't reach out and get connected.

The truth is that collaboration creates prosperity, and I'm not just talking about financially. I'm talking about prosperity in every dimension of life. Health, love, relationships, all of it. Collaboration is truly being connected to others and being in community – that's what creates prosperity. We've lost this in our culture. We have so much of the silo mentality. We need to create community.

I created this program with the intention of having a support group and a community. You're not just going through this book alone. We're going to actually create a community out of this as well. We already have a community growing, and it's awesome. There's so much value in creating community. It's harnessing the power of being part of a team. How many of you have been on a team of any sort? It's amazing how it feels to work together as a team. It's fun, it's powerful, there's so much energy. Napoleon Hill actually wrote in his book, *Think and Grow Rich*, when two or more are assembled there becomes in inherent third person. *The Bible* says this, too. There's more power. This is the mastermind concept.

What Lynn Twist was able to notice is that certain communities that practice sufficiency – they live off the land, they live with each other, they support each other – there is no fighting or possessiveness. It's a completely collaborative arrangement. Imagine what our world would be like if this was the mindset. I remember Dennis Waitley asking, "How would we need to shift our mindset so that we could have no prisons?" Because there are cultures in some parts of the world that have no prisons. It's very powerful. There are communities that exist that have this practice.

Creating sufficiency

There are several steps to creating sufficiency. What Lynn talked about in her book is that it's necessary to ***generate, distinguish and make known, not only to ourselves but to others, the power and presence of our existing resources and our unique contributions***. We have to be willing to get out of our individuality, figure out what we each have to offer, what are our resources that we can contribute, and share it with others - get it communicated. It's very important to do this – we can't hold back. Everybody has to be willing to share. This is how we create sufficiency.

There's a way to get access to sufficiency and you're going to do a very powerful exercise. First, you'll need to answer the following questions. Write at least three things for each question.

> What are you passionately committed to?
> What do you love about your life?
> What do you love to do and enjoy doing?
> What are you really good at?
> What accomplishments are you most proud of?
> Who do you admire and proudly associate with?
> What are organizations that you are proud to be or have
> been a part of?

So you can get to know me a little bit more, here is my list:

I am passionately committed to:
- Ending chronic disease on the face of the planet
- Empowering leaders to lead people gracefully and elegantly
- Empowering my four boys to be dynamic, happy and responsible men

What I love about my life:
- Being a coach and empowering people to transform their lives
- Being a father of four wonderful, amazing boys
- Making wonderful friendships with so many wonderful people

What I love to do and enjoy doing:

- Teaching, coaching
- Dancing salsa
- Being physically active – yoga, basketball, skiing, hiking

What I am really good at:
- Taking complex information and translating it into intelligible language
- Leading and guiding organizations into becoming champions
- Speaking

Accomplishments I am most proud of:
- My four boys
- Graduating from grad school at UCLA
- Having gone to med school for 3 years
- Transforming my life and my health, since 1995
- Being a published author

People I admire and proudly associate with:
- Marty Taub, who mentored me as a speaker since 1996
- Joe Harjung, my best friend since second grade
- Mike DelCampo, who taught me how to dance salsa since 2001

Organizations I am proud to be or have been a part of:
- River City Speakers, my Toastmasters club

- Sacramento Hispanic Chamber of Commerce
- Cottage Housing, a program that empowers the homeless in Sacramento

In the live seminar, I pair people up and they share their lists with each other. Then, they ask "How can we support each other?" It's a wonderful way to get to know people.

Since you're reading about this here, my invitation to you is to begin to interact with people in your life from the context of sufficiency. Start by asking one or several or all of these questions. You'll be amazed at what happens! People will think you're so interesting and such a great conversationalist. And, you will begin to have wonderful and meaningful conversations that further your lives.

I did this work with an organization called Cottage Housing – an organization in Sacramento that is dedicated to empowering the homeless so that they can get themselves back into society as contributing members. They have a wonderful track record of success. I became friends with their CEO, Robert Tobin, back in 2004. For a couple of years, I conducted workshops to empower their participants. It was a wonderful experience. But, then in 2008, Robert called me up and told me he was in trouble and asked me for some coaching. I met with him and he shared how funding was becoming more scarce and that he had to lay off some good people. He was very worried and concerned. I helped him to see that he was operating from Scarcity. So we did some work, he read some books, including The Soul of Money, and he started to see the light. He then asked if we could impart this training to the whole organization. In 2009, we had an organizational meeting with all the Board members, the entire staff and all the participants. I facilitated the meeting. We distinguished the Scarcity conversations. We then created Sufficiency and they shared their lists with each other. After, we went through a brainstorming session and generated about 75 to 100 ideas of what could make a difference. I then charged them with creating a special sub-committee to determine which idea would make the biggest difference and then create a plan of action and implement it. Last year, in 2010, their work culminated in the "First Annual Beacon of Hope" event! It was held at the Crest Theater in Sacramento and everyone came out. It was a fantastic event. And... it raised over one million dollars!! Cottage Housing is no longer in Scarcity. They are looking to expand and offer their services to even more homeless.

Imagine if our government operated this way. Imagine if the State or any large organization worked this way. What would be possible? I used to work for the State of California and I also worked for Kaiser and there are so many talented people that are under-utilized.

It's amazing how when we start to tap into Sufficiency, we become aware of the resources that already exist. When we really think about sufficiency, if we look around, we always find what we need. There's always enough. *If we share of ourselves and listen to others, there's always enough. We're whole, complete and perfect just the way we are.* All of us. And we naturally can share our resources. I remember the book, *All I Really Need to Know I Learned in Kindergarten*. We naturally share. Inside of this context, sufficiency speaks in terms of gratitude, fulfillment, wholeness, enrichment, commitment, love, trust, respect, contribution, resilience, faith, compassion, partnership, responsibility, integrity and generosity. It's the world of being extraordinary. We are thriving! We can create this. You are evolving and you can start to step into this.

Law of attraction

When I watched the movie *The Secret*, what I noticed was missing from the movie is that the secret really works only if it's in the context of sufficiency. It doesn't work if it's inside the context of scarcity. Remember, the context is decisive. We have to create the context, first.

Like energies attract – we have to focus on what we do want, not on what we don't want. What we do want in terms of a higher purpose is really most compelling. To change our reality we have to change our thinking and our speaking.

We can practice the three steps of the Law of Attraction – they are:

Number one, to **ask for what you want**. And the powerful thing is to ask inside of your higher purpose. What does God want me to do? That's the powerful question to ask.

Then to **believe**, to believe completely, that this is what you want. If you want your health and ask for your health, energy and vitality, you have to ask for it and believe that you can actually have it. You have to believe that it is possible. Anything is possible. Your body can be altered, you can create energy.

Thirdly, you have to **prepare yourself to receive** the gift. You have to do the work and lay the foundation down so you can actually receive it. There's a funny story about someone who was trying to use the Law of Attraction to attract a mate, she wanted a partner in her life. Her friend came over and noticed that her closet was completely full, that her dog slept on her bed so there was no room on the bed for a partner, and there was no room in the garage for another car. So she needed to clear out her closet, have her dog sleep on the floor and make some room in the garage. She did that and soon after she attracted a partner in her life. You have to prepare to receive.

Now that we've created this new context of sufficiency, what is a game worth playing for you? What would you like to create for your health, your fitness, and for yourself? As you're present to this, write a few things right now. What would be worth playing for? What would make a difference for you? What would you like to have? What would you like to create? There is no right or wrong answer.

Declaration is very powerful. You'll need to work with a committed friend or partner for this and declare what it is that you want as an affirmation, that this is what you are creating for yourself. For example: "I am free! I am joyfully active in my life!" Come back to these declarations over and over. Remind yourself what your declaration is and what you're standing for.

"To know and not to use is not yet to know."

Your mission, should you choose to accept it:

1. Practice giving up your statements of scarcity – let them go.
2. Then practice sharing your sufficiency list. Ask people questions such as "tell me what you love about your life?" Talk to people like that and you'll get to know people a whole different way. You'll have incredible conversations with people.
3. Thirdly, practice the Law of Attraction and state your affirmations daily.

I close this chapter with a quote from Marianne Williamson. This was also used by Nelson Mandela in his inaugural address.

"Our deepest fear is not that we are inadequate, our deepest fear is that we are powerful beyond measure. It is our light, not our darkness that most frightens us. We ask ourselves, "Who am I to be brilliant, gorgeous, talented, fabulous?" Actually, who are you not to be? You are a child of God. Your playing small does not serve the world. There is nothing enlightening about shrinking so that other people won't feel unsure around you. We were born to make manifest the glory of God that is within us. It is not just in some of us, it is in everyone. As we let our own light shine, we unconsciously give other people permission to do the same. As we are liberated from our own fear, our presence automatically liberates others."

CHAPTER 3

SECRETS OF THE FIT MIND

Here's the warning for this chapter. This chapter could bring up a lot of stuff for you. It's perfectly normal and natural if it does happen. If you hold on to what you think you know, it will limit you. This section is about letting go of what you think you know. Let go of the attachments to what you think you know. One of my favorite authors, Dan Millman, said, "Life is not suffering, it's just that you will suffer as long as you hold on to your attachments until you let go and just go for the ride." Do not hold on to your beliefs. We're going to shatter some beliefs. Do not believe or get caught up in anything that I say. It's about really staying in a beginners mind. Anytime that we get upset or stressed it's because of our perception and our reaction. It has nothing to do with anyone or anything else.

Yet, we naturally tend to point the finger of blame. We're go to explore the deep-seated blueprint about how we got to be the way that we are around our health. By the way, it applies to every area of your life as well – it applies to relationships, money, work, career, everything. You will find yourself being in a wrestling match with yourself. Here's the great part of this. The other side of this wrestling match will be a full and amazing liberation - liberation from the constraints of the past that have been holding you back for so long. That's the opportunity. The Chinese word for crisis is composed of two word symbols. One is danger, the other is opportunity. It's interesting that in Eastern cultures they view dangerous situations as a risk and also as an opportunity.

Let's start by examining the current blueprint. We all have a blueprint, it's just like any kind of building or any edifice; there is some blueprint for the construction of that building. Our blueprint is ingrained in our subconscious.

One of the things that I've been fascinated by is how our brains really work. If we really look at how we function as a human being, we think we're operating fully from our conscious mind. We think that what we're doing at any given moment is determined by our conscious mind, but it's not. Research in psychology shows that 90% of how we function is actually being determined by our subconscious (60%) and unconscious mind (30%). Only 10% is determined by our conscious mind.

We have to recognize that what's going on in our

***subconscious mind is really running the show, since
it's the major stakeholder.*** The unconscious mind is the
HeadMaster and runs the body, but the subconscious mind
is all the patterns and little voices. That's what's running the
show and we're not really aware of it. It determines the limits
of our effectiveness. We constantly try to make changes. We
say things like, "I am prosperous!" And your little monkey
says, "Yeah right, think again." If we don't get agreement from
the subconscious, guess who wins. It takes a lot of training
to overcome the subconscious. There needs to be a lot more
work involved. If we just make a statement once and the
subconscious tells you it's not true, it's not going to happen.
There are so many conversations we have with ourselves
that are so well-ingrained, and it determines the level of our
effectiveness. We need to identify the blueprint first, and then
we can actually have a breakthrough by going past it.

We're going to dismantle the old blueprint and then create
a new blueprint. This will take some work on your part. The
purpose of this section is to distinguish the pre-existing
blueprint for your health, then we'll blow it up, and then we'll
create a new blueprint. I call it the Fit Blueprint. It's a different
level of consciousness that we're going to construct.

The Old Blueprint

As a university professor of Psychology, I have come
across many theories and explanations of what shapes
our personality, our characteristics, our traits and our

behaviors. There are entire courses offered in each of these different perspectives – such as social psychology, behavioral psychology, and several others. One of the fascinating things I have studied in relation to human psychological development is how we come to shape the view of who we are.

Our self-concept basically answers the question "Who am I?" for which we may have lots of different answers. We can answer that question from several perspectives. For instance, I could answer the question "Who am I?" to describe my physical self, my personality, my social self, my character traits or my skills and abilities.

To discover where this sense of self arises, neuroscientists are exploring the brain activity that underlies our constant sense of being oneself. The medial prefrontal cortex, a neuron path located in the cleft between your brain hemispheres just behind your eyes, seemingly helps stitch together your sense of self. It becomes more active when you think about yourself (Zimmer, 2005). The elements of your self-concept, the specific beliefs by which you define yourself, are your "self-schemas" (Markus & Wurf, 1987) which are mental templates by which we organize our worlds. Our self-schemas – our perceiving ourselves as athletic, overweight, smart, etc – powerfully affect how we perceive, remember, and evaluate other people and ourselves. These self-schemas that make up our self-concepts help us organize and retrieve our past experiences in order to interact with our current situation. But more importantly, these self-schemas help us to determine how we are going to act in anticipation of the future. A simpler way to think about this – *we are constantly using our past experiences to create an anticipated view of what's up ahead on the road*. These self-schemas help us live into the future. This is what we do.

I'll give you an example. In 1992, I was working for Kaiser and had just taken the hospital through the accreditation and licensing process with the Joint Commission for Hospital and Healthcare Organizations. It's a big deal. Every three years it was a comprehensive inspection of the entire hospital and you would go through an amazing amount of work to prepare for this. I had just completed this; it was an amazing experience, I had three years of work to do in six months and had to hit the ground running. I had to make sure all the policies and procedures were completely overhauled, have meetings, put in long hours, it was a tremendous amount of work. And, I did a really good job. About a week and a half after the whole thing was done, Vivian, who I reported to and who was a no-nonsense type of person, called me and tersely told me to be in her office in five minutes. What do you think went through my head in that moment? I started living into the future thinking that I was in trouble. Her office was just down the hallway and that five minutes suddenly became very long. I get to her door, knock, and she sharply tells me to come in and have a seat and I'm thinking, "Oh man, this is it." I can visualize the blood dripping from my neck and thinking it was over. And she says, "Ruben, I have to tell you, you did a really good job on the accreditation. There's a conference for all the Quality Managers and since you're one of them, I have to send you. You're going to Hawaii. Now get the hell out of here!" So in that moment, what was the future I was living into? I went through the wringer and now I'm going to Hawaii? Hawaii then became the future I was living into – going to Hawaii in two weeks! Unbelievable!

How do we construct these self-schemas? It's really very simple. We make decisions about ourselves, about others, and about life from every single experience. We'll say things like "I'll never do that again!" "I'll never trust _____ again!" We've all had these kinds of experiences. These decisions, therefore, become wired into our brain as a protective mechanism to enable us to survive. ***Neuroscientists have determined that we fire the same pattern of neurons when we are asked to recall a past experience as when we are asked to discuss an anticipated similar experience.*** Is it any wonder then that we tend to repeat the past? We're actually wired to do so. This is the process of conditioning. Our future becomes fairly predictable because of all our experiences, decisions, and the creation of our schemas. But what if we could re-wire our schemas? What would be possible if the limitations of all our restrictive past decisions were somehow re-wired so that the future could truly be a blank slate? Anything. Anything would be possible. There would be no limits! Are you ready to create this? This is what we're going to do.

Now let's delve into how we got to be conditioned. Psychology tells us that our results are determined by our actions. What determines our actions are our feelings and emotions because we're emotional human beings. Do people buy things emotionally? Absolutely. People take action based on their emotions and feelings. Our feelings, however, are determined by our thoughts. Our thoughts and our patterns of thoughts dictate how we are going to feel. We respond to our thoughts with our emotions. But there is still a deeper level. The pattern of our thoughts is actually determined by our programming and conditioning. There is a pattern of how we've come to learn things and experience things and actually create a whole network of beliefs. Those beliefs actually create our whole programming and conditioning. So our belief system is at the underlying core of it all.

When we start to look at our beliefs, we can examine how we came to believe a certain way. That belief system then leads to a certain set of thoughts that correspond. These lead to a certain set of feelings that correspond. These lead to a certain set of actions that correspond. These lead to a certain set of results. When we start to look at the results of everything that we have in our lives, it's all based on this whole process on how we construct our beliefs, our thoughts, our feelings, our actions, and our results. That's how it all works. When we start to look at this it all becomes rather fascinating because we can start to unravel the blueprint and find out what's at the core.

We're going to start to look at how we're conditioned – how

we learned our beliefs and behaviors. There are three levels of learning - visual, auditory and kinesthetic. That's how we learn everything. We learn what we hear verbally, modeling from what we see, and kinesthetically from what we experience. We're going to start off by looking at this blueprint from these three aspects; the belief systems that we created based on what we heard, what we saw, and what we experienced.

By the way, a corresponding book for additional reading, is *The Secrets of the Millionaire Mind* by T. Harv Ecker. It is a fascinating book that applies to every area of your life.

Verbal

We're going to start with verbal programming because it's probably the easiest one for us to relate to. What were some of the statements that you heard while growing up that stuck with you surrounding health? Anything around nutrition, exercise or anything.

"Clean your plate! Eat everything on your plate. Chubby is so cute! You're not fat - you're just big-boned. You're lucky to have food on your plate. You're a big girl so you shouldn't be running. You can eat whatever you want. There are children starving in China. You better eat it before your brothers get home. Shut up and eat. You cannot leave the table until you eat that. You can't have dessert until you finish your vegetables. If you're really good you'll get a treat. Waste not, want not. You're not smart enough. It's been a hard day, let's go get a treat. Be seen and not heard. You're a lot of work. You're ugly.

Your siblings are smart, but you have common sense. Fat people are ugly. You don't need a lot of food."

Consider that the reason that memory is so indelibly ingrained is because you heard it a lot and it stayed with you. The way we work as human beings is that when we hear something over and over again, that conversation is very easy for us to remember. What we do is then create a belief about ourselves relative to that conversation. The belief can be something like, "I'll never.....", "I'll always.....", or any version of this. We construct a set of beliefs that correspond with that conversation. What is the corresponding belief that you constructed based on what you heard? We all do it, and we do it in an instant. What were the beliefs that you constructed about yourself?

Examples: "I don't deserve better. If I work really hard I'll go far. If I don't work hard I will fail. It'll be a lot of work. No one could love me. I'm not good enough, I'll never fit in. I'm weak. I'll never be thin."

Having these beliefs at the foundation has had an impact. If you look, you'll start to realize that the belief statement that you've had about yourself has had an impact. It has limited you in a particular way. There's always some impact. What's been the effect on you in your life?

To give you an example, I'll share with you about one of my clients. The conversation that she heard growing up from her father was that she only looked good from the neck up. She never forgot that. The belief statement for her was that her body would never be attractive. The impact was that she ended up with diabetes, extra weight, complete aversion to exercise, and pain. She looked gorgeous from the neck up – she took care of her hair, her makeup was impeccable, but her body was a whole different story. Look for yourself to see what that impact has been.

Growing up, I heard that I had to eat everything on my plate, so my belief was that I had to get every bit of food that I possibly could to survive so I'd eat all the leftovers, eat everything possible. Then, the second conversation that came out of that was that I was a human garbage disposal. That became a part of the background that really affected me later on when I injured myself and I defaulted to all the things that I didn't like about myself. That started to impact me because I started to eat everything I saw – I didn't waste anything.

An audience member shared that what she heard was "one day you're going to be fat" and she then became morbidly obese. She constantly heard that one day she'd be fat, and since mom said it must be true, then she became fat.

Verbal is probably the most recognizable form of conditioning for us because we remember hearing things. Now we'll delve into the other two segments, which are modeling, which is what we saw, and also the specific incidents, which is the kinesthetic. We want to use the same process.

Modeling

Let's look at things that we've seen. They don't necessarily have to be with our parents, they could be from a variety of different experiences in our life. But they tend to be from our parents. It's interesting that when it comes to our health habits, we tend to be very much like one or both of our parents or completely the opposite. It's rather fascinating how we tend to be one or the other. Sometimes we got to a point in our adolescence where we actually rebelled against our parents. That tends to happen as well.

For me, I remember being an adolescent and watching my father gain more and more and more weight. I got very angry with him and started to resent him because I'd admired him when I was much younger. I'd go with him when he went to play tennis at the LA Tennis Club and he was playing with all these famous tennis players, and he was a stud. He was amazing. I thought the world of him and then I watched him just fall apart. It really had an impact on me. The belief that I created was that I better never let myself go. I'll never let myself go like that. Then I ruptured my Achilles in 1990 and I let myself go. Finally, I had to face myself in 1995 and realized that I had completely let myself go, just like my father. I had to deal with myself and that was a powerful impact for me.

Go ahead and look for yourself, what did you notice? What did you see growing up?

Here are a couple of examples:

A female audience member comments on how her dad was very athletic and exercised a lot but her mom never did anything. So what was the belief system that you gained from that? "That men exercise and women don't." What's the impact? "I didn't exercise." She said that she sometimes did, but it became more like a novelty. Not something that she did every day but something that she tried every once in a while. Then, it became more specific – "Adult women and/or moms don't exercise." She said that she actually played tennis for awhile but it seemed very frivolous so she told herself that she didn't deserve that.

Another audience member said she had a different experience. Her parents had a grocery store when she was growing up and all the kids were taught to manage money and count the money at the end of the 12 hour day. "I remember my mom being very frugal." They were considered middle-class but her mother was ultra-frugal and she identified with those habits. So the belief she created was that "there isn't enough." She had her years of lavish spending, but overall she is very frugal. Because of that she went into the financial business and she's very good at what she does. It's interesting that something positive came out of the belief that there wasn't enough because that impacts other areas of your life. What's the impact of the conversation that there's not enough in the area of your health? "I have come to believe that it's going to take forever for me to have a healthy body. And, that there's not enough time to focus on being healthy." What we do, in some areas of our lives, we will construct a negative belief and we'll compensate and still make it work in our favor. However, that conversation is still there and it will negatively affect other areas of our life. We can have some areas of our life work fairly well, you can actually make it work for you. In your instance you had the conversation, "It's not enough" work for you in terms of becoming a financial expert and managing money very well. But that same conversation affects every other area of your life, including your health, and that's where there's been a negative impact.

What did you see? What were the beliefs that you created? How has that affected you? The invitation is to look at what's held you back in terms of your health.

Here's one of the interesting things about how we work as human beings. There are things that are in the way for us, and it's very uncomfortable to really try and deal with it sometimes. We don't want to deal with the ugly or nasty stuff. So what do we do? We develop a strategy. One of the strategies that we have is that we turn every negative into a positive, and we start looking at the positive side of things. Then we don't deal with reality. We don't look at ourselves in the mirror. And we don't deal with what's really held us back. It's just a strategy that we have – it's a survival strategy. Consider that this is an opportunity for you to deal with the reality of what's held you back. It's not an easy concept because we don't naturally want to do that. We protect ourselves. We have lots of protections and strategies.

Experiences

Now let's take a look at the third aspect of how we've learned in creating our blueprint. Now we'll look at specific incidents. Kinesthetics – the real deep emotional stuff. This is the stuff that really hits us hard, especially at the emotional level. There were some specific emotional incidents that influenced you. Focus on what was painful, uncomfortable or nasty. It's those kinds of things that have really affected us and impacted us. I'll give you a couple of examples.

One was from another participant the first time I did this course. She was, I think, 54 years old and she had been wrestling with her weight her entire life. She remembered that she was about 19 or 20 years old and she went to the YMCA because she was really committed to getting started with exercise. She was going to go swimming and she started getting changed and there were two other gals on the other side of the locker room that she could hear talking. She heard one of them say to the other, "Oh. I didn't know they made swimsuits that big." That devastated her to the point that she never put on a swimsuit again. The belief she created about herself was that she was completely deplorable. She made up all kinds of things about herself based on what she heard. For her, it was a very deep, powerful, emotional incident. And it impacted her for all those years.

We all construct amazing beliefs about ourselves.

Something will happen and we come up with all kinds of stories and interpretations about ourselves in that process. And it can be from a variety of different things. It can be from something totally unrelated to health.

One that I'll never forget was from my 4th birthday party. My mother comes out holding the cake with the four candles lit, the room was dark, my family was there, and they were all singing Happy Birthday. It's time for me to blow out my candles, I close my eyes, take a deep breath, then I open them ready to blow out my candles and my 2 year old brother had just blown out my candles. Everybody thought it was funny and cute, and it was, but I was 4 years old. I looked at my mother wondering if she was going to re-light my candles and she didn't. I was taught to be very quiet and respectful as a child so I didn't dare say anything. But in that moment I made up a whole series of beliefs – "My mother doesn't love me. I'll never get what I want. I'll never get my dreams to come true. I'm not good enough." The impact affected me in so many different dimensions of my life. By the way, I did have a conversation with my mother a few years ago. I told her that there was something I needed to share with her about my fourth birthday. She was shocked that I could even remember that far back and I told her I could remember it like it was yesterday and I told her the whole story. I told her that I had to apologize for resenting her for over forty years and making her wrong for not re-lighting my candles. She didn't remember the incident at all. So I apologized, told her

I knew that she loved me and told her that I loved her. My mother, up until that point, had never told me that she loved me. But she said the words to me, "Thank you for sharing this with me, Ruben." That was a profound connection with my mother. That's all I needed to know. By the way, I do have my four birthday candles – Aaron, Matthew, Gabriel and Joseph. Those are my four boys.

There can be some specific things, some powerful incidents that have occurred in your life. From that, write down what beliefs you created for yourself and how that has impacted you.

Strategies

What you've developed at this point is a pretty good map of your blueprint. You've got a view as to what you heard, what you saw and what you experienced that shaped who you've gotten to be today, what beliefs you established for yourself and the impact. What's interesting to look at now is that we develop a series of strategies based on our beliefs. Strategies that I'm referring to here are methods of surviving life. We have a consistent pattern of being able to survive life based on our belief system. We want to look at some of the major strategies. Generally, it's either fight or flight. That's what we tend to do.

Below is a list of commonly used defense strategies. You may recognize a few of them. Put a circle around each of the strategies that you utilize on occasion. Circle any that apply for you then put a box around the five most common and put a star next to the top two. There is usually a pattern of strategies. It's interesting to look at. We all have our own unique pattern.

Commonly Used Defense Strategies:

1. Loss of humor
2. Playing dumb
3. Endless explaining and rationalizing
4. "I'm helpless" – poor me!
5. Withdrawal into deadly silence
6. Withdrawal from negotiation/confrontation
7. Sudden onset of illness
8. Confusion
9. Sudden fatigue
10. Acting crazy – temporary insanity defense
11. Intellectualizing
12. Eccentricity
13. Being too nice
14. Trivializing with humor
15. Inappropriate laughter
16. Sour grapes – "I didn't want it anyway"
17. Self-deprecation
18. Taking offense
19. High charge or energy in the body

20. Needing to be right

21. Wanting to have the last word

22. Flooding with information to prove a point

23. Teaching or preaching

24. Rigidity – "I'm not willing to change"

25. Denial – "There's no problem"

26. Cynicism

27. Sarcasm

28. Making fun of others

29. "It's just the way I am"

30. Being highly critical

31. Blaming others

32. Hearing only what I want to hear

33. Counterattack

34. Holding a grudge

35. "I'm already aware of that"

Adapted from "How We Choose to Be Happy" by Rick Foster and Greg Hicks

We respond to every set of circumstances with actions – a set of strategies. As human beings we have common processes and strategies that we employ. We have more in common than you might think.

Blueprint settings

Now we can start to look at the blueprint and what it's set for. The blueprint is a lot like a thermostat, it's an automatic adjustment. If the temperature gets too hot, a strategy is employed to get the temperature back down to where it should be comfortable. If the temperature gets too cold, then another strategy is employed to get the temperature back up to where you're comfortable. This is what we do. We use strategies to get us back to where we're comfortable.

There are three aspects of the blueprint to examine.

The first aspect is what you are currently doing. What is it that you are currently doing, not doing, or avoiding that contributes to your health and fitness not working as well as you would like it to? Your strategies should give you insight to that because we use the same strategies over and over again. For instance, you might be highly critical of certain foods or diets. As a result, you then avoid eating certain foods. This is the part that requires you to be brutally honest with yourself. This is where the truth shall set you free. You may not like it, and I promise you it's not pretty. Take some notes on this below.

What am I currently doing, not doing or avoiding that contributes to my health and fitness not working as well as I would like? (strategies)

Based on what you're doing, not doing, or avoiding, there is a resultant impact. Next we start to look at the impact based on what you just revealed about what you heard, what you saw and what you experienced. How does that affect you? You can summarize that really quickly. What we're looking at is how this blueprint keeps you in a certain place in terms of your health and fitness. Take some notes on this now.

What is the impact on me? How do my actions affect me?

The third aspect to look at is how your blueprint impacts your attitude about yourself. What's the impact on your self-concept? You could be withdrawn, you could be in denial. What's your little monkey consistently saying about you? That little monkey is on his soap box and has got his monologue going. What's it saying? This is how you view yourself. This is at the core of it all. Take some notes on this now.

What has been my view of myself that has been adversely affected?

Consider what's probable and likely to occur – is that we'll continue to repeat our actions and have the results that we've been having. We'll continue to view ourselves the way that we have. If life were to go the way that it's been going, this would be the likely story of how it would continue to go. But this is not what we're committed to, right?

Dismantling

Now we dismantle the old blueprint. There are four dimensions to look at. Once you see this, your life will never be the same. First, there are events that occur. Second, based on what happens we will construct some beliefs. It's automatic and we do it at the drop of a hat. Third, based on those beliefs we will adopt a whole set of strategies, which we've already started to look at and examine. We establish strategies for survival so that we are consistent with our beliefs. Fourth, based on these strategies we can examine the impact based on how we then create our habits. Our habits become sustained over a long period of time, those strategies get employed over and over and over again. Our bodies are simply a demonstration of our habits.

A bodybuilder gets to be the way that they are because of their habits. Have you ever known a bodybuilder? Did you ever ask them how long it took for them to get there? It takes years. Someone didn't just show up at the gym and three hours later they walk out with massive amounts of muscle. It doesn't happen. It takes years of consistent dedication.

Model for conditioning

Here's the model for understanding how we condition ourselves at a subconscious level. There are four major parts. First, events will occur. These are what we hear, what we see, and what we experience. Second, we will then create a set of beliefs relative to the experiences. "I'll never..." "I'll always..." etc. Third, we develop a set of survival strategies to help us stay safe (refer to your list). Fourth, we'll develop a pattern of habits consistent with our beliefs and our strategies. This entire process leads to what we call in Psychology as our "perceived reality." We then set up our Reticular Activating System (RAS) in our brain to screen out anything that is contrary to our "perceived reality." The RAS then readily identifies and selects information to verify our "perceived reality."

To give you an idea of how the RAS works – Let's say you are interested in purchasing a new car, a BMW. As soon as you make that decision, you'll begin to notice every BMW on the road. I'm sure you're familiar with this. That's your RAS in action.

The RAS continues to look for evidence to substantiate that all your beliefs are in fact true. "I'm not good enough" so the RAS will look for evidence to prove that I'm not good enough. This becomes what is called a "self-fulfilling prophecy" and is inherently a part of being a human being.

However, there's an old song, *It Ain't Necessarily So*. This belief structure we have created is all based on things that happened way back when. You were younger. It's not the truth so we have to split the reality of the events from our beliefs. If we separate the events from our beliefs, what is possible? Anything! We can create a new belief. The events just end up being the events, and we can construct any beliefs that we want. We don't have to hold on to those old beliefs, we can let go of them! Yay!!

Reconstruction

Now, we can construct a new blueprint based on a new level

of consciousness. ***Consciousness is actually observing your thoughts and actions so you can live from true choices in the present moment rather than being run by the programming from your past.*** This is what we're out to do – raise the level of consciousness.

I want you to examine the pattern of the consciousness that you've had up to this point. We're going to construct some new fitness files. These are some ways of thinking and acting that are present for the fit consciousness. It's different from unfit consciousness. What we're talking about here are levels of consciousness. Don't take any of this personally. There are different levels of thinking and it's really about thriving versus surviving. Examine the patterns for yourself. Place a checkmark next to the ones that you see for yourself that you have been operating from the unfit consciousness.

Number one - unfit consciousness believes life happens to me. How you can tell this is operating is that you have experiences of blaming, justifying or complaining. When you look at your health in terms of exercise, nutrition, all of it, if this is what you notice for yourself then place a checkmark next to this.

The difference is that fit consciousness believes, "I create my life."

Number two – unfit consciousness *says* they want to be fit but are inconsistent in their action. They *say* they want to be fit, they *say* they want to be healthy, but their actions don't measure up. Fit consciousness is truly committed to being fit and is consistently in action.

Number three – unfit consciousness focuses on obstacles, problems and issues, whereas fit consciousness focuses on opportunities.

Number four – unfit consciousness resents fit people. There is the presence of jealousy, envy, cynicism and/or skepticism. Fit consciousness actually admires other fit people.

Number five – unfit consciousness associates more with other unfit conscious people. It's just the law of attraction. Fit consciousness associates more with other fit conscious people. Like-minds attract.

Number six – unfit consciousness is smaller than the problems. You can tell because there is a sensation of being overwhelmed and burdened. Fit consciousness is bigger than their problems. They expand their capacity to take on bigger problems.

Number seven – unfit consciousness is poor at receiving. You can tell if you deflect praise and support. Fit consciousness is excellent at receiving.

Number eight – unfit consciousness mis-manages time well. They are unorganized and spontaneous, especially in regards to health and fitness. There is often an attachment to being spontaneous. Fit consciousness manages time well.

Number nine – unfit consciousness lets fear stop them. They keep running into the same challenges over and over again. Fit consciousness takes action even in spite of fear. The definition of courage is taking action even in the face of fear.

Number ten – unfit consciousness thinks they already know. Other people tell them they are opinionated and cynical. Fit consciousness is constantly open to learning and growing.

Number eleven – unfit consciousness eats reactively. They frequently get themselves into a state of being famished and then eating. Fit consciousness actually eats proactively. Meals and eating are planned in advance.

Number twelve – unfit consciousness views exercise as a burden. They always find lots of reasons not to exercise. Fit consciousness views exercise as an opportunity.

Fitness files

Below are your Fitness Files – these are your affirmation statements. You want to focus on the three that are most important to take on for yourself. If you've looked at all your patterns of your unfit consciousness you want to focus on the corresponding affirmations. The affirmations are:

1. I create my life.
2. I am committed to being fit.
3. I focus on opportunities.
4. I admire other fit people.
5. I associate more with other fit people.
6. I am bigger than my problems.
7. I am an excellent receiver.
8. I manage my time well.
9. I act in spite of fear.
10. I constantly learn and grow.
11. I eat proactively.
12. Exercise is an opportunity.

With your partner or support person, declare this statement, "I am fit and I will be fit for the rest of my life!"

"To know and not to use is not yet to know."

Your mission, should you choose to accept it:

1. Say your Fitness Files to yourself frequently.
2. Continue to distinguish your old blueprint. Things will continue to come up for you, keep working on them.
3. Continue to say to yourself, "It ain't necessarily so"
4. Practice declaring your new fitness files
5. Practice new behaviors consistent with this mindset.

To complete this section, I'd like to share something that I wrote:

Metamorphosis

When its time arrives, the caterpillar moves to a distant branch and begins to spin its cocoon. The cocoon is the safe haven for the caterpillar to undergo the process of metamorphosis. Once the cocoon is completed, the caterpillar doesn't just change like a tadpole becomes a frog – reabsorbing its tail and growing its legs. No. The caterpillar must undergo a complete meltdown. The entire caterpillar literally dissolves into a mass of cells – a liquid goop. Once the meltdown is complete, certain specific cells, called imago cells, which contain the "image" of the future butterfly, begin to differentiate and organize the goop into an entirely new life form, a new structure – the butterfly! Once this process is completed, the butterfly must now emerge from the cocoon. To do this, it must create an opening so that it can wriggle out of the cocoon. Interestingly enough, the longer the struggle to emerge from the cocoon, the longer the butterfly will live. After the butterfly has emerged, it must gently open its wings and dry them out. Then it is ready to fly!

For us as human beings, we can potentially go through several "metamorphoses" in our lifetime. The process is just like that of the caterpillar becoming a butterfly. Once our "time" has come where we begin to recognize that our lives need to radically change, we begin to separate ourselves so that we can create our "cocoon" – our safe haven. We may even have several of them. This is where we can allow ourselves to experience our "meltdowns" and get to "nothing." We become essentially unrecognizable, even to ourselves. Once this happens, we can then begin to identify the image of what we wish to emerge as – a new life form – a complete transformation! We then begin the work of constructing ourselves consistently with this new image. But, we still need to emerge! And this is the struggle. If we stay focused and endure, then we can truly fly and endure as a new butterfly – a new life!

Ruben J Guzman, MPH 2008

SPECIAL SECTION:

RELEASING EMOTIONAL BLOCKS THROUGH HYPNOTHERAPY

I got a chance to meet Brianna Mitchell and sit down with her and talk about what she does. I was very impressed by her background and her program. One of the things I've noticed for myself in working with clients over the years is that sometimes there are some deep-seated emotional blocks to weight loss. I've noticed for myself, since I've gone through hypnotherapy, that it's been very beneficial. I'm a firm believer that a lot of different modalities can sometimes help with a lot of different perspectives. Sometimes I've referred people to hypnotherapy and it's been very beneficial for them. Brianna is a member here at our church and she conducted her program and I knew I needed to talk to her. I really like her approach and her methodology because it's very positive. It's not about dredging up all of the ugly stuff from the past. It's a very positive and enlightening type of process and it's very nurturing. And I thought that it was the kind of positive thing that I would like to offer because I know sometimes I can only go so far in the things that I do in terms of behavior management and coaching and sometimes hypnotherapy is a very useful tool. Brianna is a clinical hypnotherapist and I'm going to give her a chance to introduce herself and let her tell you about her background. She is also living proof, as I am, and I think it's important to listen to people who are living evidence of what they are talking about because they've used this and have been successful. Brianna has lost a tremendous amount of weight already and she continues on her path and she's done a fabulous job. Without any further ado, I'd like to introduce Brianna Mitchell.

My name is Brianna Mitchell and I'm a clinical hypnotherapist and I have a practice in the Roseville area. I'd like to get started by sharing a little bit about my story and how this worked for me. What happened for me is that I started having weight become an issue in high school. I was at a point in my life where all these things I had learned about – affirmations, making positive changes (I actually got to go to this great teen training program when I was twelve so I starting learning some powerful skills when I was young). So what happened was that I started making all these wonderful changes in my life, and then when I was fourteen I got raped.

From then on I got really afraid of life and really afraid of other people. And that's when the weight started coming on. I had never had a problem with weight before then and I started getting bigger and bigger and bigger. I've done different diets over the years. The first was an all protein diet where I lost weight but it wasn't really healthy at all and I felt sick. I got off of it and instantly all the weight came back on. I did some healthy ones, in fact I started coming to the church here and did a fat flush and was feeling really good and all of a sudden just stopped doing it. And then I'd do another one and feel good for awhile. I knew what I should do in terms of eating, but the problem was that I wouldn't do it. The better my life started getting – I got into a better relationship, I started making improvements in my life, started having better things go on with my kids, and the better my life was getting, the worse my anxiety and fear was getting, the worse my weight was getting. You'd think it'd be the opposite. Things are going well, my weight should be going down, but it was the opposite. What I got to is that it was really a deep-seated fear because of what had happened when I was fourteen. Everything in my life was going great when I was fourteen and then it crashed down. So my subconscious mind had this huge fear that this was going to happen again and I was protecting myself from it happening. Until I did hypnotherapy this was the only thing that helped me break through it. I was able to get to the subconscious fear that was driving me because I was also sabotaging myself in other ways beyond weight as well. The better my life got the more anxiety I got and I put on more weight.

I'm going to draw a circle here to show a demonstration. This little top part represents 5-10% of our mind that is our conscious mind. That's the part of our mind that's reasonable, logical, all the memory you can think of in the moment when I asked you, it's your school learning part of your mind. The big part down here, the 90-95% though, is your subconscious mind and unconscious mind. That's the part that controls your breathing, your heart rate, digestion, all the bodily functions you don't have to think to make happen. It's also the part that every memory of your life is stored in. Everything down to when you're one, two, three – all the things you can't remember now, your subconscious and unconscious mind remembers. It's where our habit patterns lie, and our blocks and obstacles. So what happens is we go through life and we start building up positive and negative experiences in the subconscious mind. They start building up and you might have completely forgotten about it. Say you are six and the first time you have to stand in front of class and give a presentation, kids being as they are made fun of you and you felt embarrassed and awful and you never wanted to do that again. You might have completely forgotten being six, until you're thirty and your boss asks you to give a presentation and all of a sudden your palms get sweaty, your stomach feels sick, you're nauseous, and you don't know why because you don't remember being six. Your subconscious mind does. We go through life and a block or an obstacle or a negative belief can be completely dormant until something or someone enters your life that reminds the subconscious mind of something that happened a long time ago. Your subconscious mind is so powerful, so you want it to be your ally, not your adversary. And for so many of us, it's our adversary.

When the conscious mind is relaxed, we can get to the subconscious mind and actually start to remove some of these blocks and obstacles. Once you remove those, then you can create space for the positive beliefs and the positive things you want in your life and bring balance. I work with my clients to bring balance to all aspects of their lives, not just weight but to enjoy your life, sleep better, bring stress levels down, really focus on all the joy that we really want in life. I analytically knew what had happened to me and I knew I was protecting myself analytically but until I got to the subconscious level it didn't change or shift. Basically, none of us are heavier than our subconscious mind wants us to be. That's really the key. Another secret dieticians don't tell you is that you're not just what you eat, you're also what you feel. Your emotions are a huge predictor of your weight, just as what you're eating. That's how you can have all this knowledge about what you can eat, but you really have to bring the emotions in to balance and work through the blocks that are stopping you. So that's where we get stuck.

I brought some music and we're going to have an experience because a lot of people don't know what hypnotherapy is or have misconceptions. When I work with clients individually I work with your specific blocks, your specific obstacles or whatever you crave. I can help so the cravings for sweets or salty foods or whatever it is that you specifically crave loses its power over you. For me, my drug of choice was ice cream. One of my clients, his was steak. He hadn't had any for a long time after working with me, and after he did he said it was like admiring a fine painting. He enjoyed it, but he didn't want it much anymore. That's what happens with this process. The foods that used to hold power over you lose their power.

Brianna then led us through a guided hypnotherapy exercise.

Anybody want to share any experiences or anything about that? The techniques that I use specifically are very empowering and they are based on that your own inner being knows how to correct the problem, knows where the blocks are and how to get rid of them. I just facilitate that process. Really, it's very empowering. A lot of times, my clients, their own answers will come to them, their own epiphanies, their own wisdoms about the situation. Actually the teacher that I went to school with for the techniques I learned was very much in line with Unity. He's incorporated a lot of things from the East and the West and really put them together. Sessions usually last a half an hour, I do them at my office in Roseville and can even do phone sessions if you don't live close.

Audience member: Is it possible to be shown the reason why you're overweight?

A lot of times, yes. Sometimes a specific answer will come to people, sometimes not. But they can still work through it whether they know or not. I also work with people who've had some severe trauma and the nice thing is that we can work through it without reliving it, which is very healing. I had one client who couldn't remember 20-30 years of her life and we could work through it without reliving it. And she actually had some good memories come back to her, but not the traumatic ones.

Audience member: How does this work for a woman who has used weight to shield people and keep them away from her?

Until you change what's in the subconscious mind, if you keep being afraid or fearful of what happened back then, it's a protection. And even if you don't need that protection anymore, your subconscious mind keeps it there just in case. So that's how this process really helps heal that. For me it was a huge protection. The better my life was getting, the more I was afraid and I was afraid of being vulnerable by stepping into my power. I felt that if I did that I'd be even more vulnerable and more unsafe so I really needed to protect myself. Basically your subconscious mind views your weight as the solution, not the problem. A lot of times the techniques I use build your strength and power so if you were in a situation that was hard or that you were afraid of, all of a sudden you know how to handle it. Or your intuition or gut feeling would be there and you wouldn't allow yourself to keep doing the same pattern. A lot of times we do need to learn that strength so if that same situation is in front of us, now we can react very differently. It's a whole tiered approach because weight is related to so many different things. It's an addiction like any other addiction. I work with lots of different addictions, and food is one of those things. It's learning how to step into your strength and how to get past the fears and use the tools that each of our own inner wisdom has. We really can draw upon it, we just have these fears that are blocking us from accessing it.

Thank you Brianna!

Brianna can be contacted at www.aproventheory.com.

CHAPTER 4

THE ENERGY MODEL

Now, we're going to look at how your body works as an energy system. The truth about how your body is designed. The overall design. Once you get this it will be enlightening. I promise you. It is quite extraordinary to go through this conversation. We're going to actually talk about the body and how we can create more energy by understanding the body as an energy system.

Let's now look at how we can create more energy. Would you like to have more energy? Okay, great, so we want more energy. How many of you have been looking for more energy in a pill? Or some box? Or some program? Or in some energy drink? How many of you have been looking for some type of energy solution? We're going to talk about energy and understand energy profoundly from the design principles of how your body is set up.

The third law of thermodynamics is that ***energy cannot be created or destroyed. It can only be transformed***. If we look from a scientific standpoint, if you understand anything about quantum physics or physics in general, we see that we have to be able to transform energy from one state into another form. For instance, these light bulbs have electricity going through them. The electricity is transformed into light. Therefore, we have light and we can actually see what it's illuminating. So, electricity is transformed from one form of energy into a different form of energy. We need to think about being able to do the same thing with our bodies.

Transformation – what does that mean from a scientific standpoint? It means changing the nature of a condition by altering the energy state. It's actually a quantum shift. It's no different than electricity passing through the coil of wire in between the two stanchions in the light bulb and creating light. It's a transformation. It's a quantum shift in the energy state.

We want to examine how we can do this for our bodies. And it's amazing that we actually have a system that's designed for transformation. Did you know that? I'm going to show you how it's set up. Would you like to know the set up?

The body is an energy system. Would you agree with that? It's just like a plant in many ways. Would you agree that a plant is an energy system? It is. Let's examine this as an analogy here.

Plants need a balance of five things, generally speaking - water, air, light, soil and nutrients. Do all species of plants need the exactly the same balance of those elements? No. Have you ever grown an orchid? Have you ever killed an orchid? They're beautiful and I love looking at them, but I think, "Don't give that to me. I'm going to kill it!" There is a secret to growing those things – I haven't figured it out yet, I'm still working on that one – but they're beautiful plants. And all plants don't need the same balance. Some plants you can throw water on, it grows, you don't have to worry about it, and it's fine. An orchid, however, is a delicate creature. It needs particular light and you have to mist it, and spray it and all these other things. I don't have time for an orchid! Not all plants are exactly the same.

Just as no two species of plants are the same, no two human beings are exactly the same either. Each of us has our own particular requirements.

Many years ago I was driving to Monterey and I was driving through Watsonville, which is known as the capital of artichokes. There's a fruit and vegetable stand with a hand painted sign that reads "World's Largest Artichokes". I had to stop. And sure enough, these artichokes were monstrous – they were huge! The farmer that owned that land was there. So, I asked him one question, "What's your secret?" Twenty minutes later he finished telling me the answer to the question. Here's what I got from his answer – that he had absolutely complete mastery of how to balance the elements for growing those artichokes. He had such mastery that he not only knew how to grow them, but he also knew how to adapt based on the changes in weather, the rain, the temperature, whatever the case may be. He could adapt to the changes in the circumstances.

We, as a culture, have lost the sense of mastery of our bodies. Much less even having the ability to adapt to the changes beautifully and gracefully.

What this program is fundamentally about is getting and mastering the fundamentals for your health and then being able to gracefully adapt. No matter what happens. You can change gracefully and still have fabulous results.

The analogy applies to us – we're no different than the plants. Fundamentally, we're a life form, but we're a little more complex than plants. So we need other things. We need a balance of nutrients and supplements, cardiovascular exercise, strength, flexibility, stress management and rest. We need all these things to be in balance.

These are, if you will, the spokes of your wheel. It's important to have all the spokes in place for the wheel to work. There is integrity to the wheel. From an engineering standpoint we say that integrity is about having everything in its place so that it works. We need to have all of these things in place to be in balance. What most of us have endeavored to do over the years, is focus on one of these spokes but we leave the rest behind. Have you every tried to true up a bicycle wheel? It's not easy, is it? You cannot do it by focusing on one spoke. It's impossible. You have to work with all the spokes, you have to balance it out, and it takes a bit of skill and practice. You have to really work with it until you finally can get it completely true. We're going to do the same thing. That's the approach here – to actually balance your wheel of life so that it can work in all areas.

Four dimensions of energy

If we look at the human being as an energy system, the wisdom of the ages has told us that there are four distinct dimensions of energy that we have. There's physical energy, which is the context of our body; there is emotional energy, which is our feelings and heart; there is mental energy, which is our ability to think, concentrate, focus and solve problems; and there is spiritual energy, which is fundamentally our sense of purpose. Why are we here? What purpose do we have? Our vision, our mission – what difference will we make for ourselves and for others in the world? These are the dimensions of our energy. And we need to have a balance with all four.

I'm going to extend this model into a corporate setting. Let's say that you are the Senior Vice President for a major Fortune 500 company. It's Monday morning. You're sitting at your desk. You're there early, and you are watching people coming into the workplace. Here's what you know. You know that there is a lot of stress in the workplace because there are talks of an impending merger. None of the vacancies that have occurred in the last six months have been filled. Everyone is having to put in extra effort and do the work of all the people that have left. There were a series of layoffs, the company is down about twenty five percent in revenue, and there's a lot of tension in the workplace. You can feel it. That is what you do know.

You're watching your Human Resources Director walk through the door. But, here's what you don't know. She had a fight with her spouse the night before. And, yes, it was about money again. She didn't get a good night's sleep, she had a tough time with the kids in the morning, she got scratched by the dog, almost hit two cars, only had a cup of coffee and a doughnut, and God knows the last time she exercised. Given that scenario, what is her physical energy? It's pretty bad, you can see it. She's lethargic, haggard, she looks tired, and it's first thing Monday morning! Given that as the foundation, what's her emotional energy? Positive or negative? You can bet your bottom dollar, it's negative energy. What is that going to fuel in the organization? Criticism, cynicism, skepticism, resignation, gossip – all those kinds of things. By the way, gossip will kill an organization! Given all this, what's her mental energy? Is it sharp or is it dull? You better believe it's dull. Gallup polls show that forty seven percent of the American workforce is mentally disengaged. Nineteen percent is actually actively disengaged. They're surfing the internet and playing solitaire. Given all this, what is her spiritual energy? Is she truly aligned with the mission and vision of the organization or is she there to survive and get a pay check? She's in survival.

Now when it comes to organizational performance you can bring in a motivational speaker; you can do the fire and brimstone meetings as well; you can try to impose guilt on people, but how long do you think that's going to last? Until the doughnuts are gone – that's it. It's short lived. If we recognize from an organizational standpoint and an individual standpoint, we have to address all of these energy levels, and it begins with the physical. If our physical needs are not being met, nothing is happening. We're in survival. Some companies are starting to get the picture. They're starting to put gyms in the workplace, they're starting to empower people to actually go workout, but they're still missing the boat because they're not addressing what's really missing, and that's lifestyle. That has to be addressed. They're just putting icing on top of mud thinking it's a cake underneath. It happens all the time. The only way we can improve performance is to really get down to the bottom of it, start really scraping off the mud. We have to look at all four dimensions of energy. That's what it takes. It's going to take that for you individually. Can you imagine what it's going to take for an organization? It's a lot of work. And, yes, this is one of the things I do.

Energy model

Now, let's talk about the energy model. What I've got here is the body as a car – this is my ideal car.

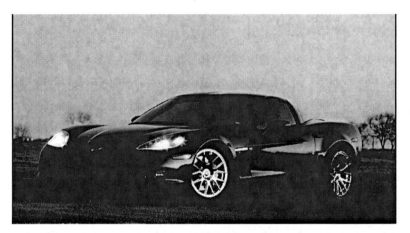

Your body can be anything you want it to be – you can be a broken down, old, beat up Volkswagon Beetle with rusted parts, blown out windows, and no muffler. Or, you can be a souped-up, beautiful, high-performance Corvette, or anything else you want. The choice is yours. Your body can be transformed the way you can transform an automobile. You can transform metal into anything. That's one of the things I learned from my father. My father was a machinist and we used to build things. We'd take raw wood and raw metal and we'd build all kinds of things. You can shape things into anything you want if you've got the imagination. If you create a plan, you can do almost anything. It's amazing. So, your body is like a car. I've drawn up a model of a car, and this is my crude, simple yet accurate model for health and how the body works.

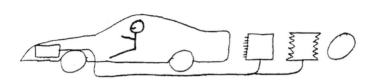

If your body is like a car, there's a part of your body that drives the rest of your body. What would be the part of the body that drives the rest of the body? Generally speaking, it's your brain. There's a collective consciousness in the rest of the body, but generally speaking the brain drives the rest of the body. I call this your HeadMaster. This is really at the unconscious and even subconscious level, but mostly unconscious. Your HeadMaster is in charge, it runs the show; you have no say in the matter. Isn't that surprising? You have no conscious say in how your body runs, but you think you do. You do not. It's as if there's another person running your body, and it's not you. How many of you have had that feeling before? I had to look in the mirror at myself in January 1995 and thought, "Who did this? It wasn't me, I didn't do this. I would never intentionally do this to myself." Your HeadMaster did it. The reason is that your HeadMaster monitors and controls 99.9% of everything that's going on inside your body. Consider the evidence. Do you consciously create blood cells? No, but your body is doing it all the time. Do you consciously digest your food? No, but your body is doing it all the time. Do you consciously create hormones? No, but your body is doing it all the time. Do you consciously adjust your hormones? No, but your body is doing it all the time. Do you consciously grow your hair? I've been trying for years, it still doesn't work!

Your HeadMaster is in charge. You are not in charge. You are in charge of one thing – you are in charge of your habits. You get to choose your habits. Based on your habits your HeadMaster will then choose one of two software programs. Imagine your body's computer has two software programs, that's all. Dr. Kolitsky told me this when I was an undergraduate, I didn't realize the significance of this back then, not until many years later. "All if life is in one of two states. Either it is surviving or it is thriving, and that's all there is." So if it's surviving, I call it the crisis software. If it's thriving, I call it the happy software.

Your HeadMaster is either surviving or thriving. You choose your habits. Your HeadMaster is basically reading the dashboard. You got to bed at 2 a.m., got up at 5:30 a.m., you didn't have breakfast, all you drank was that God-awful coffee, you didn't have lunch, you worked all afternoon, you had three handfuls of sugar, and you came to dinner and you had that big steak with all that grease, and that oily salad, and really buttery potato with dripping cheese – your HeadMaster is in survival! And God knows the last time you exercised. If those are your habits, your HeadMaster is going to be operating the crisis software.

We have to recognize that your HeadMaster is going to respond based on your habits. The HeadMaster is all-knowing, all-seeing, and cannot be fooled. It's like Sister Mary Lenore, my HeadMaster in eighth grade. You could not get anything past her. Nothing gets past the HeadMaster. You may think you can fool the HeadMaster, but there is no fooling the HeadMaster. If you try something for two days, then go back to the way it was, don't think your HeadMaster is going to change. It changes only based on consistency. You have to train the HeadMaster to adapt to your habits based on the good habits that you set yourself up with.

In survival, here's what happens – the sum of all of our habits is negative and the Head Master then has to do whatever is necessary in order to survive. It will have the body at dis-ease. The body is not at ease. This is the source of all disease. It's when your body is running in crisis mode over, and over, and over again. That's the source of heart disease, diabetes, cancer, and osteoporosis. You name it, that's it. It's because the body, fundamentally, is stressed.

The happy software is run only when we take good care of our body and our habits are positive. In that situation the Head Master is able to thrive. That's when you can build muscle, have strength, have energy, vitality. All those things can happen; they're possible.

Research experiment

We're going to do a little experiment, I need a volunteer.

Ruben: What's your name?
Leah: Leah

R: Leah, would you come up to the front for a moment, please? Leah, thank you for being willing to do this experiment with me. First I want to reassure you that there will be no physical harm to you whatsoever. This is a simulated experiment, so I want you to play along and go along with it as if it's actually happening for you.

L: Okay

R: You can act out anything you want. Are you a good actress?

L: Pretty good

R: Very good, just use your imagination. Let your imagination run wild. It's a two part experiment, here's how it works. Each experiment is one week in duration. Here's part one. We're going to take a trip down to Southern California. How's that sound to you?

L: Sounds good

R: Sounds good? We'll see about that. Leah, we're going to take you down to Southern California to a very special location. It happens to be the lowest land elevation in all of the United States. Do you know where that happens to be?

L: Desert?

R: Desert? Good guess. Have you every heard of a place called Death Valley?

L: Yeah...

R: Oh good, you have. So this is where you're going to go.

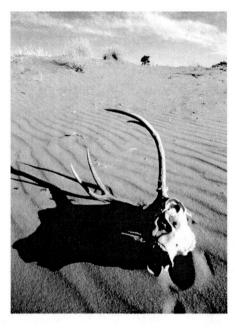

You're going to spend an entire week there. Here are the conditions. You're going to spend an entire week on the desert floor, you'll have a tent – a little one, you'll have a four day supply of water, and a four day supply of food. That's it. And you're going to spend seven days here. By the way, it's August. The temperature on the ground floor has been hitting about 121/122 degrees. It's a little hot. You like the heat?

L: Uh, not so much.

R: Knowing that you're going to go there, what software program do you think your HeadMaster selects?

L: Survival

R: You're going to run the crisis software. I want you all to get this because without even going there, just the thought of it is enough to trigger a hormonal cascade in your body. How many of you know when you're about to step into a stressful situation and you feel it in your body? We don't actually need to have the experience. Just thinking about it is enough to start the stress reaction. Leah, what's your plan to survive this?

L: Well, I don't drink enough water anyway, so the water thing wouldn't be a problem, I'd make it stretch out. And I skip meals, so I could probably get by. Stay inside during the day, come out and cool off at night, I guess. Just lay low.

R: OK. Let's fast forward now. It's been five days. Five long, hot, sweltering days. The low has been 101. High has been 123. There's no electricity, no cell phone, nothing. It's just you. You can't go anywhere. You're stuck there. What's the status of your water and food supply, and how are you doing?

L: Not good. I would imagine that I'd probably be pretty clammy, sweaty, dry mouth, feeling dehydrated, lethargic.

R: Absolutely. And your food supply? How much food have you eaten?

L: Probably most of it. Maybe a small amount left.

R: How about your water supply?

L: Probably pretty similar. I've used more than I would have liked to, I imagine. Trying to keep a little bit of something.

R: So you're just really lethargic.

Research Team, what's happening to Leah? She's in survival, so what's happening to her metabolism? It's definitely down. Metabolism is her body's ability to take food and synthesize it and convert it to something new. Her energy is down. Adenosine Triphosphate is a chemical in the body that we can measure, so that's definitely down. We're not synthesizing ATP. What about her sensation of hunger? Five days in. She's not hungry. At this point the brain says, "Famine! No sense being hungry." Starts to shut it off. Do not believe the myth that your weight problem is because you overeat and that you need to suppress your appetite. Especially if they have names like Dexatrim. Do you love to eat? Yes, right? See, it's normal, isn't it? You're designed to eat. You're not designed to starve. Now when you start to shut off the hunger sensation it's because there's something wrong; you're in a famine, you're starving. She's now in this situation. The hunger switch flips off.

What is Leah's capacity to store food as fat in this state? The capacity to store food as fat rises significantly. Based on various research studies – you can take a group of athletes, very lean male collegiate athletes, 6-10% body fat - the kind that can sit down and eat a 24" pepperoni pizza by themselves and not gain an ounce of fat. Have them go through their regular day, training, eating, exercising, everything, and have a standardized meal at the end of the day. Like spaghetti, meatballs, vegetables, salad, garlic bread – the whole bit. They have been able to calculate that only 6-10% of that meal would get converted to fat, even though the fat content of the meal was much higher. That's all their bodies needed. Then have them go through another day, same routine, exercise, training, all of it. Except for one thing. Do not allow them to eat the whole day, until the final meal. They eat the same standardized meal. Now, 28-32% of that meal gets taken up as fat. What is the difference? The state. They were in survival, starvation, they were in crisis. It doesn't matter what the label says. How many of you are stuck on reading what the label says? How many grams of fat, how much of this, how much of that? You can let go of that now. It doesn't matter. What's more important is the state that your body is in. If your body is in crisis, no matter what the label says, you're going to store more of it as fat. If your body is thriving and doing well, you will only store what you need as fat. Isn't that amazing? Did you just have a light bulb go on? I hope so.

By the way, cattle ranchers have known about this process for decades. They get more money for the beef if it has a high amount of marbling, which is intramuscular fat. For the last couple of weeks before taking them to market, the ranchers will starve the cattle for a day, then feed them lots of processed grain, then starve them, then feed them, and so on. This is how they increase the fat in order to make more money. Amazing!

Now, Leah, it's day seven, you've been really having a tough time. We're going to end this part of the experiment. We're going to take you to the Palm Desert resort where we're going to get you rehydrated. We've got a team of doctor's waiting for you. We'll take care of you, pamper you, get you back to normal in a couple days.

Now we're going to part two of the research experiment. We're going to the airport. What you'll get to do now is select any tropical resort in the

South Pacific that you would like to go to, carte blanche, for an entire week. You're going to get your own personal massage therapist, your own personal chef, you're going to have the time of your life because you're going to be able to do anything you want for an entire week in paradise. Where would you like to go?

Leah: St. Lucia

Ruben: OK, that's in the Caribbean. So you're going to the Caribbean. This is what your bedroom window looks like.

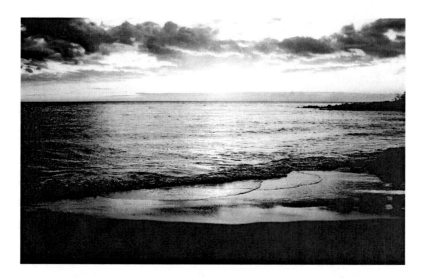

Knowing that you're going there, what software do you think your HeadMaster selects?

L: Happy!

R: Amazing. By the way, just the thought of going

someplace really fabulous – how many of you notice when you've booked your vacation to a tropical resort, how many of you notice a shift in your health and your vitality? It's amazing, isn't it? Just the thought of going there is enough. That's when your vacation really starts, the moment you book it. We're going to fast forward to day five. What have you been doing? What's it been like?

L: Relaxing on the beach, yoga, lots of massages, spa treatments, nice, healthy breakfasts, long, leisurely walks, naps – lots of naps.

R: Great! She's definitely running the happy software.

Research Team - What's happening to her metabolism? Definitely goes up. What happens to her energy level? Also goes up. What happens to her sensation of hunger? Goes back up to normal levels. Because she's got Guido ready at a moment's notice to prepare her anything she wants. So it goes up to normal levels, she gets moderately hungry, she gets something to eat, she doesn't get to being starving, she's always got enough to eat. She's just fine. What happens to her capacity to store food as fat? It goes down. By the way, folks, this is the only way it goes down. The only way it goes down is to actually run the happy software. You must run the happy software, otherwise the body hoards the food and converts it to fat.

Question: Does the quality of the food you're taking in have a bearing on whether your body is in crisis mode or thriving?

The quality does matter, but it's not the most important thing. We will discuss this more fully when we get to the chapter on fat reduction, and we'll talk about survival food. However, the state we're in is the most important thing. A really interesting example is top level athletes. For instance, one of my best athletes, Matt Moser. I coached him from when he was ten years old. Amazing athlete, great swimmer, fabulous water polo player, got a full ride scholarship to Stanford in water polo. He was one of those guys that could sit down and eat a 24" pepperoni pizza all by himself and not gain an ounce of fat, and he was about 6% body fat. He could do that any time. He was a machine in terms of how he burned fuel. So it depends on a lot of factors, including, what's the state of your car? What's the state of your body? How high-performance is it? If it's not at that level, then the quality will make a more significant difference. At his level, he could get away with just about anything. Could he do that for the rest of his life? I don't think so. By the way, that's why many NFL athletes have had some serious health problems after they retire, because they continued to eat at a same level as when they were competing. More of them are starting to understand how to eat more effectively now because the older ones had some serious health problems. This is the most important aspect to get – *your body functions based on the state in which it is in. Everything else hinges on this aspect in the model. I want you to understand that the state that your body is in drives the results. Are you in survival or are you thriving? What software is your body running? That's the critical question.* What we have to be able to do is learn all the significant aspects to running the thriving/happy software. Do you want to be able to run the happy software and keep running it? That's what we're out to do in this program.

CHAPTER 5

BEYOND DIETING

We've established that, as human beings, we suffer from insanity, right? The insanity of doing the same things over and over and expecting different results. How many of you have been on more than one diet? If you've done more than one diet, and failed, you're suffering from insanity. There are so many diet programs, diet tapes, diet shows, diet doctors – there's all this stuff that's out there about diets. There are so many different diets. We suffer from insanity because we clearly haven't figured it out, so we need to take a radical and different approach. Remember Einstein's quote, "The significant problems we face cannot be solved at the same level of thinking we were at when we created them." We created the problem, and then we lodged it into our subconscious. We didn't consciously create our problems, we subconsciously created our problems. So we created our problem and we have to find a way to actually release that problem. That's what we're out to do here.

The purpose for this section is to review the energy model that we talked about earlier and to talk about how the fuel system of your body works. In any energy system, if you understand the fueling of the energy system, it gives you power to understand how the energy system really works and you can work with it as opposed to against it.

Most of you actually drive an energy system named an automobile. You don't have to know everything about the inner workings of the automobile, but you do need to know how to fuel it. Most of you would not open up a can of tomato juice and put it in your car. It wouldn't work so well. So you know you have to put in the right kind of fuel to have your automobile work. That's common sense.

We're also going to develop a very specific 3-prong approach. It's very simple and we'll talk about mastering the priorities in those three areas. If you're looking for the magic bullet, the quick and easy fix, it's not happening. I want you to have the correct information to be completely and effectively empowered to reduce body fat.

It's not your fault

Part of what we don't realize is that our bodies are actually designed to store fat when we are in the state of survival. Think of the following scenario:

Let's say you are a Native American Indian living in the hills of South Dakota five hundred years ago – long before the white man arrived. During the spring, summer and fall seasons, there is an abundance of food available – berries, fruit, vegetables, grain, everything!

But then winter hits! There's a lot of snow. It's really cold, and you find a cave for shelter. You may have some food stored up. And, you bundle up, huddle up and try to stay warm. You're not doing a whole lot – just waiting for the snow to melt and spring to re-emerge.

Physiologically, in this state, your brain registers that you are in survival. It will also shift your brain chemistry to unconsciously seek out **SURVIVAL FOOD**. These are the foods that get converted more readily to fat, which is the best form of survival fuel in the body. Survival foods are what you crave and seek out – sugar, salt, starch and fat! This is so you can make it through the winter. And, it's designed to be a temporary phase.

However, our culture has created a permanent survival "winter." People are constantly under stress and they are unconsciously seeking survival food. And the problem here is that once we start consuming survival food, our brain keeps us seeking out more survival food. "It must still be winter." The fast food and other restaurants know this rather well. That's why their food is laden with sugar, salt, starch and fat. Once you get started, your brain flips the survival switch ON and keeps it on, and keeps you coming back! It's not quite an addiction, but it is a vicious trap!

So it's NOT your fault that you have gained weight. It's just the trap of the design. You've been stuck in it. What's important now is to recognize how you've been trapped in the survival mechanism of the design.

When we're in survival, our metabolism goes down, as does our energy level. Our sensation of hunger goes up initially for a short period of time then it goes down. Because what the HeadMaster will say, over time, is that you shouldn't be hungry because it's a famine, there's no food. It will then automatically suppress the appetite. We've come to believe the myth that people are overweight because they overeat need to suppress their appetite. It is a complete myth substantiated by people that own companies like Dexatrim. How many have ever been on a medically supervised, amphetamine diet? It's completely based on the myth that you are overeating and need to suppress your appetite. We're all designed to eat, we enjoy it, and there's nothing wrong with having an appetite. But we've come to believe that there is something wrong with being hungry and enjoying eating. From here on out you have complete license to enjoy eating – you have my permission! How many of you now have a sense of relief? It is perfectly normal to enjoy food. When we're in crisis mode, we suppress the appetite, and that is unhealthy. It is healthy to have an appetite.

What happens to the capacity to store fat when we're in

survival? It goes up. That is how the body stores fat. When we're running the survival program, when we're under stress - it doesn't have to be the physical stress of not having food, it can be emotional stress – when the Head master says we're under stress, we store food as fat. Fat is the ultimate survival fuel. There was some research done on the survivors from Auschwitz, the death camp. In June 1945, they rescued the survivors and they were actually able to determine that they still had body fat. Even though they were visibly just skin and bones and could not walk, they still had body fat. Their muscle was gone. The body will consume the muscle first and save the fat for last. It's the most condensed fuel that we have. Consistency of our habits, therefore, poor or positive, is very important to take note of.

When we run the happy software, all the things we just talked about get reversed. Metabolism goes up. Energy goes up. Sensation of hunger goes up to normal levels. The capacity to store food as fat goes down. That's the only way it can go down. We have to run the happy software and then we're at ease.

Diets don't work

Diets can never, ever, ever work. How many of you have ever reduced calories? How many of you have ever been under 1200 calories a day? Here's what happened when you're under 1200 calories a day. – you were running the survival software. Your Head Master thinks that it is a famine and recognizes that it is not getting enough fuel. Then it sets itself up to store anything that you eat as fuel – mostly as fat. How many of you have been caught up in reading the number of calories on food labels? Say goodbye to this, you don't need to do that anymore. It's not about the calories. It's about the state your body is in. Your body will respond to the state it's in. Diets can never work because the Head Master selects crisis and the capacity to store fat increases.

Here's what you do lose when you go on a low calorie diet. You do lose water, and you do lose muscle. It is possible to lose a dramatic amount of pounds doing it that way. You could lose a lot of weight. It's possible. But it's not healthy. When people focus on the scale and what the number on the scale says, they're missing the point about how their body actually functions. They aren't losing fat, they're actually setting their body up to store more fat and convert more of the food into fat after they get off the diet. I had a client once who was 62 years old and she counted more than 60 diets that she'd been on. She gained more than a pound and a half from each.

Anybody know how the cattle ranchers increase the value of meat? Get more marbling in the meat. You know how the ranchers do it? They feed them for a day, they starve them for a day, they feed them for a day, they starve them for a day. It increases the intramuscular fat. Therefore it increases the value of the meat at the marketplace. The animals are also fed corn, which is unhealthy for them and therefore it gets passed along to the people that are eating it and it's unhealthy for them as well. This is the same mechanism of how diets are set up. They are destined for failure. Every single one of them. They can never, ever, ever work. From this point onward it's never going to be a calorie restricted diet, you'll never have to worry about counting calories again!

Fuel system

Now we're going to have some fun with understanding the fuel system. Here's the diagram below.

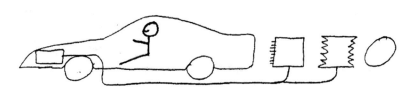

We've got the car, we've got the engine, and we've got the main fuel line. There are three tanks that we have available to run on. These represent the three different types of fuel that we can potentially burn.

The first tank is glycogen. Glycogen is the human form of sugar. You cannot buy it at the store, it is not prefabricated. Your body has to manufacture it. We are the perfect manufacturing plant for glycogen. You can buy the sources for glycogen. The best sources are whole grains, legumes, vegetables, fruits, nuts and seeds. Those are your best sources of food that actually get converted to glycogen. We store glycogen in our liver and locally in the cells. There is only a limited supply; you cannot store an infinite amount. We have a fuel level of glycogen and we have to replace that glycogen over time because we use it. You burn glycogen very slowly when you sleep, which is a good thing.

Complex carbohydrates are your best source of glycogen. I'm going to make the distinction between complex carbohydrates and simple carbohydrates. Complex carbohydrates have a molecular structure of lots of different branches of sugar molecules. Because the complex carbohydrates have lots of different multiple linkages, our body works better at being able to utilize those so it can more slowly clip these off and reformulate them into glycogen. Simple carbohydrates are one, two, sometimes three molecules of sugar. These kinds of carbohydrates are too simple. The body can't break these down into glycogen because of their size and shape. The chemical nature of those carbohydrates is such that the body has to do something with it very, very quickly. It's too hot of a fuel. It's almost like having nitroglycerin in a regular car. Refined sugars act like that. Maltose, lactose, glucose, sucrose – those are all refined sugars. What happens is the body has to secrete insulin to deal with it because it's too refined of a sugar and it can't utilize it or break it down more slowly. It has to deal with it right away so it secretes insulin and the insulin has to shuttle the sugar out of the blood stream. Guess what it's going to do with it? The body is so efficient and doesn't waste anything so it stores it as fat! So the next time you look at that doughnut or that chocolate bar or that sugar-coated cookie, think what's happening in your body. Your body is storing it as fat.

Do you know how much sugar is actually in your blood? Most people don't do the calculation. I did this with my son the other day. For the average human being, the amount of blood in the body is about 5 liters. The amount of sugar that you should have in your blood is anywhere from 80-100 mg per deciliter. When you calculate that out, it ends up being about one teaspoon of sugar for your whole body. That's it. One little teaspoon of glucose for your entire body. Do you know about how many teaspoons there are in a can of Coca-Cola? Sixteen. It's very easy to flood the system. When we get low on glycogen, the HeadMaster is watching the fuel level and evaluating the fuel level of the glycogen tank. Once your glycogen level gets down to the bottom, the HeadMaster tells you that you're running low on fuel. Now in an automobile, you run out of gasoline, what happens? You stop. As human beings, we don't do that; we actually have a reserve fuel tank. The HeadMaster says, "I am running low on fuel, shut off the mail fuel line. Go get emergency fuel." So it turns the valve. Kind of reminds me of my dad's 1972 Chevy truck, he still has it. It's got an extra fuel tank that you can reach down and turn a valve to access the second fuel tank.

We shut off the glycogen fuel line completely, but we still need emergency fuel. We have two choices — fat or protein, those are the other two fuels that we have. Where are we going to turn for fuel? You'd love to go to fat, wouldn't you? Life would be easy. Just don't eat, burn all the fat, life would be beautiful. But we go right past the fat and start running on protein. We start burning muscle protein. It's not a very efficient fuel, but we'll burn it. And it's not very good for productivity.

One of the things that happens in athletes, for instance, is we start practice at 4:00, by 5:00 we're hitting the training sets pretty hard and I start seeing some faces that aren't feeling so good. What do you think my first question is? "When did you eat last?" And here's what the usual answer is – "I had a glass of orange juice and a pop tart for breakfast." And that's been it. What do you think I do at that point? I kick them out of practice. At that point, anything else that they're doing is counter productive. They're breaking down the very muscle I'm trying to help them build so they can get stronger! At that point it's futile for them to try and continue on anymore. Anorexics run an extremely high risk of heart disease and heart failure. This is because they're digesting all the muscle in the body including the heart muscle, which causes their heart to become much weaker.

When we starve ourselves we run into what I call the Red Zone. This process of getting into the Red Zone and then starting to burn muscle protein typically takes, on average, 4-5 hours. Three meals a day, six hours apart is enough to put you into the Red Zone three times each day. "Three square meals a day" does not work. Have you heard that you should eat your three meals a day and no snacking? Throw that one out the window. Biochemically, it makes no sense. Our bodies are designed to eat consistently so that we have glycogen in the tank. When we're in the Red Zone and we're burning muscle protein, anything that we take in, a higher percentage of it, is going to be stored as fat.

You're probably wondering, what about the fat? How do we tap into it and burn it? You have to understand the design. Our fat is actually a linked fuel. We have glycogen as our gasoline and fat as our oil. Do you know what type of engine uses both gasoline and oil as a fuel? Diesel. That's the setup – you're a turbo diesel Mercedes! You burn fat as your oil and glycogen as your gasoline. We have to realize that we cannot burn fat without the presence of glycogen. Conversely, if you have glycogen present, you can burn fat. If you do not have glycogen present you cannot burn fat. It doesn't work – that's just the biochemistry and the human design. It's a concurrent fuel. This is why marathon runners have fueling stations. They've learned that they have to eat, especially if they're going to run for such a long time. They need to eat on a consistent basis. It's very important.

You don't want to burn protein. If you burn protein, one of the products of burning protein is called ketones. If you've ever had a doctor tell you that you need to use a dipstick to measure your urine and make sure you have ketones in there, that's malpractice as far as I'm concerned. Ketones are the breakdown of proteins which leads to ketosis if it's prolonged over a period of time. You keep on doing that, you can ask any emergency room doctor, it gets really bad and you get to a state called ketoacidosis. This means your body is now in an acidic state. You've now changed the pH in your blood and you've put it into a negative and survival state. If you have a diabetic that comes into the emergency room in ketoacidosis, you now have a medical emergency. Therefore, in my opinion, any doctor telling you to go into ketosis, such as Dr. Atkins, is engaged in malpractice. By the way – most diabetics in this country are undiagnosed. Diabetes has been increasing at a rampant rate and it's an epidemic.

While you sleep, as long as you have some fuel in the glycogen tank, you're fine. Everything slows down so you're not burning the glycogen as fast. You hear a lot about not eating after a certain time at night – total myth. You can absolutely have a snack in the evening, and may in fact need to before you go to sleep. However, you don't want really want to eat within an hour of going to bed. There are some rules on this but we'll talk about the digestive tract and how it works a little later.

I'm going to give you some principles on how to actually fuel your body without following a restrictive diet plan. The principles I'm going to present are based on the science of how your body actually works. Consider that humans are really more alike than different. I've done enough autopsies to tell you there really isn't that much variability. Biochemically and physiologically we're much more in common than we are different.

You're number one priority for fat burning is to absolutely stay out of the Red Zone. Do not allow your body to get into the Red Zone at all, at any time. When that happens, everything negative gets triggered. It is not a pleasant situation for your body.

Cravings

Let's talk about cravings for a moment. In the afternoon, do you sometimes get a craving? Or in the evening - do you get the munchies and have to get something to eat? Here's the setup. We talked about glycogen already. The body needs to have a proper fuel level. The brain, however, does not run on glycogen. The brain actually runs on glucose. Your blood glucose level is necessary to run your brain. You need to have a small amount of glucose in your blood stream for the purpose of running your brain – about one teaspoon, remember. Your brain burns glucose. It's a different chemistry for your brain. That's why paramedics, when they set someone up on an IV, they always have a little bit of sugar in it to make sure that person does not go brain dead. If they go brain dead, it's over. So you have to have a little bit of sugar. It's only one teaspoon for your whole body, that's all you need. Not a whole lot. We have a system to manufacture all the glucose we need. We break the glycogen down and there are a couple biochemical reactions that form glucose to then feed the brain. Just enough for one little teaspoon. We normally maintain that level by eating healthy food consistently. The blood sugar level is very, very delicate. We don't need very much. If we get into the Red Zone, the HeadMaster shuts off the main fuel line completely. Now we also just shut off the capacity to turn glycogen into glucose. When we get into the Red Zone, it's a double whammy. Not only are we starting to break protein down, but we've now shut off the supply of glucose for the brain. Now your HeadMaster says, "Feed me. Feed me now or die!" And in this state the chocolate is actually talking to you, calling your name! The corn chips, the potato chips, the starchy foods – they talk to you! Have you noticed? Your HeadMaster then drives your body to a place called Sugar City or Sugar Mountain (which I found at Niagara Falls).

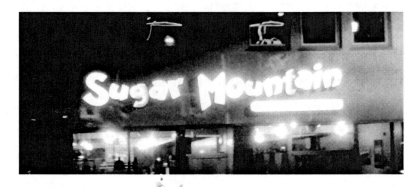

Your brain, your Head Master takes over out of survival. You have to because at that point you've cut off the supply and you must get sugar into your system in order to feed your brain. The high-glycemic index foods are perfect for that. Those are things like sugar, starchy snacks, and potato chips.

What about fasts and cleanses? There are many different types and there's a psychological aspect to those as well –

some people can handle it, some people can't. The cravings still happen and the body can still start to adjust but most people doing it start to bring their activity level way down. They have to. They bring their activity level way down so they can maintain some of the glycogen level. But people often do get into trouble doing it. I personally don't advocate that people try those.

What are the symptoms of the being in the Red Zone? Headaches, irritability, shaky, grouchy, brain stops working, nausea, desperate for food, unclear thinking, very sleepy – these are typical symptoms of being in the Red Zone.

3-prong approach

We now know how things look when they're not working. Now let's talk about how to get them to work. We're going to talk about three things that we need to do to get the fueling system to work effectively for effective fat reduction. There are three aspects. One is to improve the nutritional habits. Second is to develop consistent cardiovascular exercise. Third is to develop consistent strength training. We're going to talk about mastering the fundamentals, the basics, and get your body working in a positive direction.

Nutrition

Let's first talk about nutrition. If we understand the system and how it's set up, the priorities become very obvious. We need to have glycogen in the tank at all times. We cannot afford to go into the Red Zone. ***Your number one priority in terms of nutrition is to eat consistently. Every two and a half to three hours.*** Do you love to eat? Now you get to do it more often. Interesting, isn't it? You may be thinking that's not what you've been told. Yet, you are actually designed to eat every two and a half to three hours.

If you're a mother and you nursed your children, how often did you nurse them? Every two and half to three hours. I have four boys, so I watched the process. What happens if you do not feed your child every two and a half to three hours? Havoc! Your first 1-2 years of your life, you're set up to eat every two and a half to three hours. That's the design and that's the programming, and it works. If we were designed to eat every 6 hours, mothers would be very happy because they'd get more sleep.

Your brain works a lot better if you're eating every two and a half to three hours. Hand in hand with this is having just enough to eat. You notice that babies eat until their full and that's it, they're done. They don't nurse forever; they go until they've had enough and then they stop.

This requires a shift to being proactive as opposed to being reactive. This is where you have to start to think ahead. You're driving a car and you're going from Sacramento to Chicago – it's a long trip. You're going to have to stop along the way and refuel your tank from time to time. Are you going to start off on empty? No, you're going to start off with fuel in the tank and you're going to be proactive and put gas in the tank before you get to empty. You're not going to want to run out somewhere between Utah and Wyoming.

You have to start thinking proactively about how you fuel your body, the same way. You want to eat consistently and you want to eat enough to sustain you for the next two and a half to three hours. How much fuel that is for you is going to be individually determined. Every body is different based on your lifestyle, your habits, and your activity. If you're going to do a workout in the next two and a half to three hours, you're going to burn more fuel, aren't you? So you probably need to fuel up with a little bit more beforehand. If you're going to be resting or just lounging, you're not going to use as much fuel so you don't need to eat as much. It's thinking ahead, a difference in thinking. We will talk about the quality of your food later, but what I'm saying is ***HOW you eat is far more important than what you eat. What you eat is important, I'm not saying that it isn't, but HOW you eat is far more important.*** You need to sustain your body to stay out of the Red Zone and eat enough to sustain you for the next two and a half to three hours. It's a difference in thinking. How you approach food is like fueling a car. It's very different up here in your brain; that's where the shift has to occur. You'll have to experiment for yourself. We can make changes, but we have to train ourselves to eat a different way. It's learning what we need to eat and what is going to sustain us for the next two and a half to three hours. No counting calories – throw that out the window. You'll have to play around with this, I can't tell you how much to eat. I was actually trained as a nutrition consultant and that's what I was taught to do – develop prescribed menu plans with so many calories and intervals of when to eat. But every person is different. I could create an initial plan, but your life is going to be your life. What you do and your activity level, how your body works and how it digests, that's individual. I can give you a range – usually it's going to be between 1800 and 3000 depending on the individual. If you're an athlete like Michael Phelps, you're going to burn 4000-5000 or more calories a day, easy. Every body is different.

Your mission, should you choose to accept it, is to *start focusing on eating every two and a half to three hours, being proactive in your eating, and eating enough to sustain you for the next two and a half to three hours.* Start to experiment. I promise you this, you start doing this and you will start to have amazing energy within two weeks. I promise you. It absolutely happens every single time because your HeadMaster starts to recognize there's no more famine. The fuel line stays open and you get to burn the fuel much more efficiently and much more effectively. By the way, if you eat this way, it will raise your metabolism.

Hydration tips

Let me take a moment here to also talk about hydration. Food and water are critical to the physiological function of your body. Your body is about 65% water, and a drop of even two percent can adversely affect your energy status, put you into survival, and decrease your metabolism. Therefore, it's important to drink enough water throughout the day. Your body absorbs about one cup of water within 15 minutes. And, you are losing water all day through respiration/breathing, the digestive process, through your skin and via urination.

The most important time of day to re-hydrate is *in the morning as soon as you get up. Drink a big glass of water*. Your body does NOT need the coffee to wake up, it needs the water!

Drink a cup of water about 15 minutes before you eat. This will help to rehydrate you more quickly. You may notice that you won't feel so hungry while you eat. We usually need water more than food. You can survive 3 days without food, but you can't go more than a day without water.

You should also drink enough water throughout the day such that you are urinating every one to two hours – this would be good hydration. If you want to do this right, just drink water – nothing else. Of course, common sense applies here, don't drink a large amount of water just before going to bed. Otherwise, you'll have to get up in the middle of the night.

Cardio

The second prong is cardiovascular exercise, which will also raise your metabolism. At the cellular level, we have these little organelles called mitochondria. What they do is take fuel and convert it to the human energy molecule, otherwise known as adenosine tri-phosphate or ATP. If we set up our cardiovascular exercise correctly, then we can, over time, stimulate an abundance of mitochondria, which means you can now burn more fuel and produce more energy.

Simple stuff – here's how you do it. If you want to change your physiology and get more mitochondria, it takes 5-6 days a week, not 3. Have you heard that you just need 3 days a week for cardiovascular exercise? Throw that one out the window. Three days will maintain you where you're at. *If you want to change your physiology, it's 5-6 days per week.* How many of you were ever athletes before? How many days did you work out? Five, six or seven days a week. I rest my case. Now, it doesn't mean you have to do two, two and a half hour workouts a day.

The intensity should be what's called a high aerobic level. You want to work your way up to this. If you're not able to do this right now, that's fine. Start from where you're at and gradually move upwards over time. Do what your body will let you do. If you can only walk at a mild pace and that is enough to get your breathing going and your muscles to work a little bit more, then do that. You want to work up to the ideal level where you can breathe comfortably, but barely. You could talk, but quite frankly would rather not. Don't always believe the machines at the gym that tell you when you're in the fat burning zone. That's based on marathoners who are genetically very, very different. What they've shown is that if they're working at a low level and sustaining it for 26.2 miles, they actually then do burn fat at a higher proportion than glycogen. The "fat burning zone" is based on that research but that's not normal. This approach is about changing your physiology not what you're burning in that moment. What we're talking about here is transforming your physiology, which is building a bigger engine. How can you build a bigger engine as quickly as possible with the least amount of effort and the least amount of time? Don't pay attention to the charts at the gym. By the way, heart rate is only a secondary indicator and we'll talk about that in a minute.

You want to be working your way up to the high aerobic level. ***You want to be barely breathing comfortably and you'd rather not talk. All it takes is twenty minutes at that intensity.*** You need a little bit of a warm-up and a little bit of a cool-down. Twenty minutes. I used myself as a case control study. That whole year, 1995, I did it exactly this way. Twenty minutes, that was it. The heart rate is not what you want to focus on. The heart rate is a secondary indicator. The American College of Sports Medicine talks about this - it's is called the "perceived level of exertion." It's much more important than the heart rate. Heart rate is statistically based on a bell shaped curve but not everybody exists in the median range, so you want to work based on your exertion. Your homework this week is to get that started.

What we're talking about here is actually changing the physiology and triggering certain enzymes to kick in to actually trigger physiological replication of the mitochondria. So if you do something more intensely for ten minutes it's not the same as doing it at an aerobic level for twenty minutes. There are different biochemical factors that are involved and they work very differently. A great book to read on this, written by Covert Bailey, is called Smart Exercise. We're talking about less than thirty minutes with a 3-4 minute warm-up and cool-down.

Strength

The third prong, strength, is very important as well. What we've seen in the research is that if you combine cardiovascular exercise with strength work, you will have a multiplication effect. It's not twice as effective, it's four times as effective at changing the mitochondria and changing the physiology. It is much more effective to combine the two. Now you don't have to do a whole lot. Strength training builds bigger pistons. My favorite adage is *"growing old is not for sissies."* It's not. You CAN get stronger. Anyone can build muscle strength, it is possible to do. Jack LaLanne was a great example for us all, he lived to 96 years old and he could kick just about anybody's butt. Everybody can get stronger. I'm not saying you need to be a body builder, but you should be able to do just a few things. If you're feeding the body properly and consistently, then you can actually build the muscle protein. When we get to our strength chapter, I will detail some workout exercises with you. You want to use some simple exercises. I'm going to show you one now.

This is called a wide stance squat.

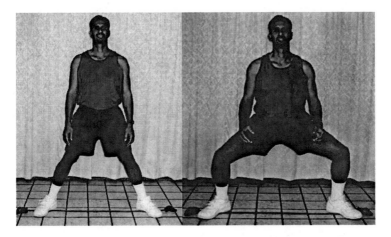

Take a wide stance with your feet, about double shoulder width apart, turn your toes out 45 degrees, keep the bottom edge of your rib cage up, bend your knees slightly. This is your starting position. You can carry an imaginary bowl of water in your hands and not spill a drop. Come down nice and slow and come down as far as you can, keeping your shoulders back. Slowly come back up. Don't forget to breathe. Your legs should be talking to you. That is the most comprehensive exercise for your lower body.

In the strength chapter, I'm going to teach you how to do a total body workout in just three exercises. That's one of them.

How do we build muscle strength? Consistency! There's the magic word again. 3-6 days a week to change your physiology. You can do those exercises every day, it's perfectly fine. The stuff you hear about having to rest a day is based on body building mentality. That's working your body to failure. Have you ever done body building before? If you work to failure you have to rest. You can't use your muscles for the next 24 hours.

Here are some exercises for you to get started. You can do squats, you can do push-ups against your kitchen counter and you'll be amazed at how much strength you build up in a short period of time. You don't have to do a whole lot. It's about consistency and the intensity is only to a level of fatigue. When you've had enough, stop.

Fat reduction profile

When we look at using all three of these prongs together – using nutrition effectively, eating consistently, eating proactively, eating enough to sustain us for the next two and a half to three hours, we're engaging in cardiovascular exercise, we're doing it 5-6 days a week, building those mitochondria, we're working to the level of intensity that is in the high aerobic range, we're doing it 20 minutes a day not counting warm-up and cool-down, we're doing strength training 4 days a week - if we're doing all of this there will be a likely scenario about how things will change in your body.

Let's say, for instance, x lbs. is your total weight. You have a certain part of your body that is lean mass, which is comprised of your muscle, bone and water. The fat mass is strictly that – fat. Your body is composed of those two main parts; that is your body composition.

Here's what happens. When you start an exercise program and you haven't been doing all of this stuff before, you start to feed your body properly, you start to exercise properly, you start doing strength work, you're doing it all. And if you're watching just the scale what can happen? It tends to go up. Why does it go up? Because you're building muscle, usually fairly quickly. What happens to the fat? It stays the same because you haven't quite built the machinery yet to start burning fat more quickly. What can typically happen in the beginning of this program is you can start building lean muscle and your fat hasn't been able to be mobilized yet and you look at the scale and see it go up. What many people do is they read only the scale. They get upset because they're gaining weight. They think the program isn't working so they freak out and they stop. This is what's called Phase One; this is very typical. Is gaining lean mass a bad thing? No, it's actually a good thing. It's important. If you broke your arm, it was in a cast, and you took the cast off, your arm would be fairly skinny. That's called atrophy. So you exercise and the arm starts to gain back its lean mass. It's healthy. Gaining weight isn't necessarily bad. You have to look at the composition. Gaining lean mass is Phase One.

In Phase Two we continue to increase lean mass and we start to decrease fat. We basically have an exchange. Total weight stays the same, and it is a little increase from what it was before. "Now this really isn't working! I'm working really hard, I'm feeling wonderful, my clothes are fitting better, but the scale isn't moving. And it's still up!" That's Phase Two, also very common.

Do not pay attention to the scale! Don't quit!

We don't gain lean mass forever, thank goodness, so we level off and we continue to burn fat. At this point, what's happening to the total weight? Now it's finally going down. And it goes down very quickly, usually, at this point. Not until then do we actually start to see the scale drop. You have to set the system up right, then you start to see a drop. This is Phase Three.

Then finally we reach a point where it's a new equilibrium. Fat levels off, lean mass levels off, total weight levels off and we reach a new balance point. But the thing is, we've changed the body composition dramatically.

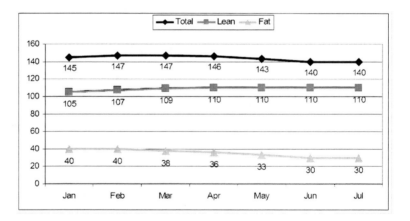

I used to measure my athlete's body composition every single month. One of my girls, 5'-9", started at 145, went up to 147 and ended up at 140. The thing was that she gained five pounds of lean mass and decreased ten pounds of fat. That's a fifteen pound differential in terms of body composition. That made a huge difference. But the total weight difference was only five pounds. The scale can be deceiving. Do not go by what the scale says.

If you go to Amazon.com, you can order your own body fat analyzer for under $35. The company that makes it is called Omron. You can get your own device. You can measure your body fat and it's a good tool to use if you really want to measure body composition.

Don't just measure total weight. You need to have four measurements: total weight, percentage body fat, your fat mass which is your total weight times your percent body fat, and you subtract your fat mass from your total weight you to get your lean mass.

There are different ways you can measure your body fat. You can use a dunk tank, which is uncomfortable for most people because you're in a swimsuit and you have go underwater, let out all your air, and hold it. The skin calipers don't work as well, that's only the subcutaneous fat. It doesn't measure all of it. This device I have is a bioelectric impedance body fat analyzer. It's much more dependable, much more reliable. When you do it, do it the same day of the week and the same time of that day. Use it under the same conditions so it becomes more reliable and more valid information. I usually do mine every Sunday morning if I'm going to do it.

Here's a chart of body fat percentages and levels of risk, because as you increase body fat we do know now that you have increased risk of cancer, diabetes, heart disease and stroke.

General body fat percentage categories

	Women	Men
Essential fat	10-12%	2-5%
Athletic	13-20%	6-13%
Fit	21-24%	14-17%
Elevated risk	25-31%	18-25%
Significant risk	32% or more	26% or more

What is the right percentage of body fat for you? There is no perfect percentage body fat. Here's how you know, and Dr. Denis Waitley calls this the mirror test. You stand in front of the mirror buck naked and when you can stand there and say "YES!" that's the right percentage body fat for you. And it feels good. When you get to that point all that matters is that you're happy and you feel your body.

"To know, and not to use, is not yet to know."

Your mission, should you choose to accept it is:

1. Practice the priorities of consistency and quantity for your nutrition.
2. Schedule time for eating.
3. Begin your cardiovascular program and don't stop. Start to figure it out.
4. Begin your strength program. Do a little bit, but do it every day.

I'll finish this section with a poem from Soren Kierkegaard:

The Possible

> *"If I were to wish for anything,*
> *I should not wish for wealth and power,*
> *but for a passionate sense of what might be,*
> *for the eye, which ever young and ardent,*
> *sees the possible.*
> *Pleasure disappoints,*
> *possibility never.*
> *And what wine is so sparkling,*
> *what so fragrant,*
> *what so intoxicating*
> *as possibility."*

Live into the possibility of being healthy and fit for the rest of your life. Begin it now!

CHAPTER 6

NUTRITION

Let's dive into nutrition. This will be a fabulous part of the entire program because we're going to talk about what you put in your mouth. We're going to cover a lot of things that are discussed in *Forks Over Knives, The China Study, The McDougall Plan, Diet for a New America, Skinny Bitch, Skinny Bastard* and other great books. I'm not going to repeat everything that's in those books. I'm going to cover some other things and give you a different framework from which to actually view nutrition. It's different. Those books will be a complimentary resource of information for you.

I'm going to present a different perspective for you. We're going to review a little bit about what we talked about last time as far as the energy model and the priorities for nutrition. And then we're going to dive into my food ladder. And yes, it's called Ruben's Food Ladder. We're going to understand food from a scientific perspective, understanding how the gastrointestinal system actually works. This is based on a lot of science and a lot of observation having done quite a few autopsies. And I can tell you having done a number of autopsies, there is a dramatic difference between the gastrointestinal system of those people that die from chronic diseases versus those who were healthy and had a healthy diet. Hugely different.

We've established that we, as human beings, suffer from a condition called insanity. We continue to do the same things over and over again, expecting different results. We continue to look for some answers to our issues, our concerns, our challenges, our problems. We continue to look for some new diet plan. How many of you have been on at least two diet plans? Most people have been on a lot more than that. We're not clinically insane. We're just insane from our practices. What we need to do is take a different approach.

We're going to establish a priority for fueling your body in a way that works with the design of your body. I'm going to submit that there is a design. Have you spent any time out in nature? Like enjoying hikes, enjoying nature and lakes and trees? You get that there's a design - a design to all of life. If you study biology you start to see the amazing intricacies of the design of every life form. In fact, there is a numerology to pinecones. There is a sequence to the spiral and the angle and the number – it's exact and it's always the same for that particular species. Do you know how many seeds are on every single strawberry? There are 200 seeds on every single strawberry, regardless of the size. There's an amazing aspect to the design of everything in our universe.

The second thing I'm out to do is to empower you to use a simple system to make positive behavioral changes in your nutrition that you can use day in and day out. From here on out we just want to make it really, really simple. Not complicated. How many of you have been in a complicated program? You had to cook this, and you had to weigh that, and you had to measure this? It's tiring, right? It's exhausting. We're going to make things very, very simple.

Each of us needs to discover our unique design. For example, you could plant a Northern California Redwood tree in a large pot in your living room, but would it grow to it's full capacity. No. Why? It's not designed to grow in your living room. But, if you were to plant it in a place like Muir Woods, it could potentially grow to a couple hundred feet. Like a plant that has a unique design to thrive and do well, so we, too, have to figure out the balance for us. How does that work? As far as I'm concerned, I do not believe that there's one plan for all human beings on the face of the planet. I don't even believe that there are four plans, like the Eat Right for your Blood Type Diet.

By the way, here's why some of those so-called diets seemingly work. Here's the reality. 90% of the American population eats absolutely horrible. You write a book that's got a halfway decent diet plan and if anybody follows it then, guess what? They're going to get better results. That's just the reality. It doesn't mean it is absolutely the truth about what you must and should eat. It's just something better than what you were doing from before. That's why any of those diet plans are popular, because they give you quick results. By the way, there is absolutely, scientifically, no correlation between the antigen- antibody response on the surface of the blood cells, which is blood typing, and a correlation to your nutritional needs based on the type of food you should be eating. Absolutely none. The Harvard School of Public Health and the UCLA School of Public Health completely decimated that book. Same thing with Atkins, same thing with the *Zone Diet*, same thing with a lot of these diets that appear. The major thinkers in nutrition in the leading schools of public health have completely shown that there is no scientific basis for many of these programs.

The major concept for this section is that ***HOW you eat is far more important that what you eat.*** Most of us have been trained to think the opposite way. Because when we think about getting healthier we think about choosing foods differently. Almost all the books that are written out there tell us what foods we need to be eating, yet they seldom talk about how to eat. What you eat is important, I'm not saying that it isn't, but it's not as important as HOW you eat. When you have the choice of going another four hours without eating or eating a bran muffin now, what's the choice going to be? Eat the muffin now rather than go into the Red Zone and go into crisis. You have to have something in your system so you keep your system fueled. Even if it's not a great choice, it's the best choice now.

So we have the body like a car and we have three fuels tanks. The first fuel tank is glycogen – the human form of sugar. The second tank is fat, and the third tank is protein. And we've got our engine which is all of our cells and our organs. Our main fuel line is connected to glycogen and fat. Can you burn fat without glycogen in the tank? No. You must have glycogen in the tank at all times, it's critical. What's the best form of food that you can eat that gets converted to glycogen? Complex carbohydrates. So any diet plan that tells you not to eat carbohydrates is ridiculous. We need to have complex carbohydrates. That's our gasoline, it's what our body runs on. The fuel gage is on this tank and this is what the HeadMaster is checking to see if you have enough fuel in the tank. We also talked about what happens when you get low into what we call the Red Zone. It takes four to five hours to get to the Red Zone. How many of you noticed that you got into the Red Zone this last week? Awareness is the first step to a transformation. What did you notice when you got into the Red Zone? You crashed, felt nervous, weak, panicked. It's good to be aware of that because we want to break that. It's really critical. When you get into the Red Zone the Head Master has to shut off the main fuel line and get emergency fuel from the protein. That's what happens when we start to break down muscle protein.

It's not good.

If you went to a doctor on a medically supervised diet they probably told you that they actually want you to have ketones in your urine, which is the breakdown product of protein. Protein degradation will result in ketones in the urine. That's what the medically supervised diets do with doctors that have no medical training in nutrition, no medical training in weight loss, no training in being healthy. They're not qualified to teach anybody how to lose weight. I should know!

We want to always make sure we stay out of the Red Zone. If we're in the Red Zone, what happens to our food when we eat? You will store a higher percentage of anything you eat as fat. The body will naturally convert it. Remember that fat is a linked fuel. Therefore, we have to think of glycogen being the gasoline and fat being the oil, so we're basically functioning as a diesel engine. We can't think of our body as being fueled by one energy source, it's a combination. We need to have a little bit of fat and mostly complex carbohydrates. ***The number one priority for health is to absolutely stay out of the Red Zone.*** For those of you who got into the Red Zone last week, continue becoming aware of being in the Red Zone, and do everything you possibly can to stay out of it. ***Plan your meals, eat every two and a half to three hours, and eat enough to sustain you for the next two to three hours.***

If you do happen to get into the Red Zone you want to eat good complex carbohydrates and you want to eat slowly.

When you eat feverishly, your body is triggered to store more of that into fat. Eat enough to get you off of that sugar problem that your brain has when you're in the Red Zone and maybe eat every 20-30 minutes to get yourself out of the Red Zone.

The American culture – work all day, work really hard, have a little bit of lunch, get home at 7:00/7:30, now you've gone 6-7 hours without eating and you're starving. You eat a big meal at a Mexican restaurant where the plate is huge – you got two enchiladas, the taco salad, the sauce, the cheese, the chips and salsa, and you've finished it all. Because you're so hungry you put it all away and that is going to get stored at a higher level as fat. The best thing to do instead is get some raw vegetables and get them in your system which will start to get you out of that Red Zone, give you a little fuel, and then you won't eat as feverishly.

If you're physically active you can get into the Red Zone much quicker. The glycogen tank is limited, remember. We only have so much fuel that we can store. If you're physically active, you could potentially deplete your tank very quickly. That's why it's so important to eat about an hour before exercise. That'll give you enough time to digest the food so it's stored as glycogen so that you have it in advance, in preparation for the physical activity. And then you want to eat within 30 minutes after exercise. That's the most critical time to refuel. Now if you've got a long set of exercise, for instance the triathletes or marathon runners, you've got to bring food with you. You've got to stop and eat along the way. You have to because you're going to be burning up that fuel. If you don't, you're going to get into the Red Zone. And in sports we call it bonking. You need consistent fuel. It's always dependent on the circumstances. It's up to you, your activity, your fueling – there are a lot of variables. You have to figure out what's right for you.

Most of us have a variety of different symptoms when we know we're getting low. We start to get hungry, and you feel hungry. That's your body telling you that you need fuel. That moderately hungry sensation is nature's way of telling us that it's time to eat. The glycogen gets converted to glucose and brain actually runs on glucose and when we get really low, the brain doesn't function so well. The second signal when we get really low, you get light-headed, you get dizzy, you get irritable. Some people actually have hypoglycemic episodes where they black out, get light-headed, or get faint. This is also the point where we start to crave things. Once you get to that point the HeadMaster says, "I need glucose and I need it now." That's when the chocolates actually start talking to you. (Audience member makes a comment about sugar being the quickest way to get sugar to the brain.) It is, but it's a very addictive process. What we do is eat the sugar, which we have to in order to feed the brain, but we realize that was really good so we want more. The whole thing is that we eat more than we really need. Our blood sugar goes way up and the brain recognizes there is too much sugar in the system now, so we secrete insulin and as we start to secrete insulin the blood sugar starts to go down. As the blood sugar goes down, the insulin goes down and now we've got low blood sugar! And now we start to secrete glucagon to increase the blood sugar. It takes a long time to re-regulate this and we drive ourselves crazy!

Digestive system

Let's dive into how the system works physiologically. We're going to take a little journey. We have a gastrointestinal system that is access for everything that we eat and drink. It all has to go into the gastrointestinal system. It's an amazing system. Incredible design.

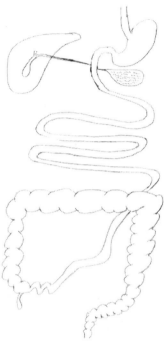

The entire gastrointestinal system is typically anywhere from 14-17 feet. That's from the throat all the way down to your anus. That's the length of it. It's pretty long, especially if you have to split it open by hand and wash it out, like I did with all those autopsies. I learned a lot about the gastrointestinal system by splitting it open and cleaning it out many, many, many times. It was quite an insightful education. As distasteful as it may sound, it was rather interesting. I could tell a tremendous difference in the pathology, the external texture, the internal texture, the folds, the color, the odor. All of it was very, very different. There were two classes. One was all the people with chronic diseases. Basically their intestinal systems were very much the same, they had a lot in common. Here's what I saw. The muscle lining of the intestinal tract, especially in the small intestine and the large intestine, the muscle lining was rather thin. It also was rather grayish in color. It did not have the richness in color. It did not have as profuse a blood supply. It also, for a lot of people, had a lot of fat attached. It was pretty slimy on the outside. When I opened it all up, what I noticed on the colons for most people was that they didn't have a lot of folds on the internal part. For most people the folds were flattened out. In the small intestine I noticed that the folds were very much flattened out, and a lot of times there was a coating of mucous on the inside. What I also noticed was that the food that was in the intestinal tract didn't clear out as easily. It was sticky a lot of the time and it took a lot of work to actually clear it out. It wasn't very water-soluble, it was more fat-soluble type food. It was stuck in there. Especially the meat. Meat does not break down very well. It sticks in the intestinal system and it's very sticky, there's a lot of fat in meat. The odor was horrible. If you weren't prepared, and sometimes we'd have a guest come in to observe an autopsy, it would knock you on your butt. In fact my first experience ever being in an operating room was a ruptured colon repair. I nearly got knocked out, I almost blacked out. I had to sit down, the nurse came over, gave me the smelling salts. It's bad. I can't even describe it. It's like the worst port-a-potty you can imagine – but ten times worse. That's what I noticed to be fairly common. That was what the gastrointestinal system in most of the autopsies were like.

I think I shared the story about the woman who was the Seventh Day Adventist. She came to the hospital, mid-70s, shortness of breath and she died a few hours later. Her intestinal system was completely different. It was no different than a healthy teenagers'. It was pristine. It was perfect. Everything looked like it was brand new. It was pink, thick, the folds were full, it was beautiful. Cleaning out the intestinal system was easy. Everything just washed out quickly. And the odor was almost inconsequential compared to the rest. She actually had a very rare heart defect where she should not have lived past the age of twenty. Clearly what she ate made a difference. She had no dairy, no meat, no caffeine, no alcohol, no tobacco, and she walked 5 miles every day. So her lifestyle was the key to her health. The evidence was there and it was undisputable. All of her organs were that way. There was no additional fat. It was quite a spectacle to behold. There is an amazing beauty to the design of a body. And when you've seen it, it's quite something to behold.

Audience question: why is it when people go in for a colonoscopy everything looks so pink and rosy and pristine? Well, there are a couple things. One is that they clean it out because you've had to be on a fast to do a colonoscopy. The difference is when somebody is alive, they have blood supply so it will be pinker. When they're dead you can see the difference because there is only a residual blood supply. This woman who was a Seventh Day Adventist had residual in the tissue that was so pink and so perfect versus the rest who die from chronic disease where there wasn't that much blood supply. Internally, when you're alive and everything has been cleaned out and you can do a colonoscopy it'll look good, but it's deceiving. Unless you start digging around you can have diverticulitis or other types of things going on. But you can't see what the effects are of the diet because you've gone through this horrible drink that's cleared everything out. It's nasty. It's very dramatic what happens to the system. It's like 100 x Ex-lax.

Let me go into how food works in the system. It typically takes about twenty minutes for food to go through your stomach. No matter what you eat. It'll be in your stomach for only about 20 minutes, no matter how much you eat. That's why you want to eat just enough to sustain for the next two and a half to three hours because your stomach will do a better job digesting that quantity of food, which is a smaller quantity. It'll start to break it down much better than if you loaded in a whole ton of food. That's one of the problems that we have in the American culture – we have these large meals, dump a ton of food in there, it doesn't get properly digested and have indigestion. The stomach can't process it and 20 minutes later it moves on through and the stomach isn't done processing yet. Your stomach can only hold so much. It doesn't stretch to enormous sizes, it's got a limit to what it can actually stretch to and after that it's going to push things through or it'll come back up.

Another problem we have with the Standard American Diet is that we tend to have a lot of processed food, meat, dairy and oil, which have a lot of calories but don't give our brain the proper stretch-receptor signals that tell our brain that we've had enough to eat. Therefore, we tend to eat more of these high calorie foods before we get the signal that we've had enough.

Your stomach is an acid bath. The purpose of the stomach is to start the digestion process intensely and chemically break food down. The acid starts to break up the chemical bonds that form the food. After the food has been in the stomach for 20 minutes, it starts to move into the duodenum. Where you actually absorb your nutrients is in the small intestine. That's the area that is the longest part of the intestinal tract. Then it goes to the colon for dehydration. Everything is more like a soup consistency in the small intestine and the colon is going to dehydrate, absorb most of the water and make it much more solid for elimination. The total process typically takes about 24 hours. Usually if you're having intestinal problems at the tail end it's usually because of what you ate the day before.

You should have about 2-3 bowel movements a day if you're eating properly. If you've got enough fiber, if you're eating consistently enough, you will have 2-3 bowel movements a day. When you're not getting bowel movements you're storing more of it. It backs up your system when you're not excreting or eliminating waste. Your body will start to become toxic and overloaded. Your kidneys, your liver and your lungs have to work harder. This will lead to dis-ease in your system. It's happening more and more because of the poor quality of the diet. The medical community will not be alarmed if you have 3 bowel movements a week. They say it's average. I say it's not even close. Are you a parent? How many times a day did you change your child's diaper? Your child was eating every 2-3 hours and you were changing a poopy diaper at least 3 times a day.

Question: The acid bath in the stomach – is it impacted by the fluids that you drink before a meal? Does it aid or hinder digestion? Here's the reality about the system and how the stomach works. A lot of people have heard all kinds of mythology out there. The stomach is designed to secrete gastric acid and it usually gets to a pH of between 2.3 and 3.2. That is very acidic. It will continue to secrete that acid no matter what you put in the system. To dilute that you would need to have something very alkaline or a lot of water. But it's not going to dilute that much of the acidic nature of your stomach. If you have too much food, it won't have enough time to break the chemical bonds of the food itself. If you eat food and then drink a ton of water after that our body will secrete more acid and then start to break food down but it won't necessarily be enough time. So it's a matter of time more than it is about the content. Now if you drink a soda, for instance, that's got a low pH to begin with so your stomach doesn't need to secrete very much acid at all. In fact, you could put a hamburger in a can of soda and it'll dissolve. A lot of people think you shouldn't drink before you eat or you shouldn't drink after you eat – that's more of a personal preference than anything. Here's something that I've noticed and it's fairly interesting. If you drink a big glass of water about fifteen minutes before you eat, you tend not to feel quite so hungry. Consider that the most important thing that most of us need is hydration first and then we need food second.

Most of the time we're thirsty and we don't even know it. I think it's a great practice to get into by starting your day with a big glass of water. The hunger sensation isn't there so much because a lot of times what I needed was a big glass of water. Your brain is 80% water so you need to hydrate the brain. Then you can eat a little bit later and you won't be as hungry so you eat just enough.

Priorities for fueling

When we look at the whole energy system we can determine the priorities for fueling your body.

As mentioned before, number one is consistency and number two is quantity. These are the most important aspects to master. Master the consistency and the quantity. It'll make the biggest difference for your diet and your health.

Thirdly we're going to talk about improving quality. That's the third priority, don't have it backwards. Most people operate with quality first and then they maybe think about consistency and quantity. Your HeadMaster will thank you if you get this right. You're going to eat about 5-7 times a day if you eat every two and a half to three hours. You get to eat! Your body is designed to eat. You get so much energy and so much more vitality, you get more productivity, more alertness, your brain functions a lot better. Literally I've told CEOs and executives, "Look, you want to raise the bar on productivity, eat every two and a half to three hours. If you get all your staff to do the same thing you will start making more money. I promise you. Because now you'll have a staff that is thinking more clearly during the day." You want to establish a rhythm and a regular schedule. As mothers, how many of you knew you needed to have a rhythm and a regular schedule for feeding your children? You did. We are designed that way from the get go. The quantity is about eating just enough to satisfy. It should keep you satisfied for the next two and a half to three hours. This will be an experiment and it's different for all of you. It depends on your lifestyle and it depends on your activity. There is no cookie-cutter plan for this. I will not even begin to suggest it for you, you will have to experiment. Every one of us is different. If I told you what I ate and you tried to duplicate it for yourself, it probably would not work because our lives are different. You have to play around with this and experiment and you'll figure it out and it will start to work.

The most important thing is to consider eating proactively and not reactively. It's about planning,

thinking in advance, always carrying something with you and always being prepared. I carry food with me all the time. I never allow myself to get into the Red Zone. You need to be prepared so that you don't get into the Red Zone and you don't falter. You need to keep your system fueled at all times.

Now, let's talk about the quality of what you eat. Here's the overriding philosophy when it comes to quality – ***simply make better choices.*** You know what they are. You just focus on making better choices – that's the most important thing. If you go out to eat at a restaurant, and if you don't ask, you don't get. So if you have the internal conversation that says, "Oh, there nothing on the menu I can eat", this is not an acceptable conversation. It doesn't work and it's not empowering. I have been in restaurants with a group of friends, and everything on the menu was either steak or seafood and that's all there was. There wasn't a speck of anything that I considered acceptable for me and I got a little frustrated. But, if you don't ask, you don't get. You have to be willing to ask and be creative. I got the waiter and I tell him that I have special dietary needs – use those words, by the way, it's very powerful. Say, "I have very special dietary needs and cannot have any meat or dairy in my diet. Would you be so kind as to ask the chef if they can prepare something for me so that I can actually eat here tonight?" Feel free to steal those words. It is an empowering conversation. When I've used this, I had the most amazing meal and everyone was usually envious of my meal. I've done it several times, in restaurants all over the country. I've had to customize and ask. Sometimes I look at the appetizers or the a la carte items and wonder if I can combine different items. Then you just ask. Most of them are actually rather excited to do that for you. The chefs get to be creative and they love doing that. So, for the quality – just make better choices, no matter what the circumstances.

Ruben's Food Ladder

I'm also going to empower you with my food ladder. This is a way of looking at food. We're going to look at it from a scientific perspective so you can understand how food actually works in the digestive system. It's not about counting calories or counting fat, or counting grams of cholesterol or anything like that. How many of you have been on diets before where you had to count points or calories? Get rid of that. Freedom from that for the rest of your life – how liberating is that? We're going to make it really simple.

Here are the criteria for understanding how food actually works in the digestive tract. When I studied in medical school and did some research on the gastrointestinal system and combining that with my autopsy experience and laboratory experience, I started to realize there are some major aspects to understanding the human digestive system. I actually compared the human digestive system to other animals. You really learn a lot with comparative anatomy and physiology. It's very interesting to look and see the digestive systems, the enzymes, the biochemistry, the physiology. It's very fascinating to look at all that.

3 factors

There are three major aspects to consider scientifically in terms of food and how it actually interacts with the digestive tract. The first one is **digestability.** This means that the food actually breaks down to a molecular level so it can actually pass through the wall of the intestinal tract and enter into the blood stream. You could eat a Cessna airplane, but it's not very digestable. It doesn't break down and it doesn't transfer into the blood stream, not very well. You may get a few molecules of metal from the shavings and that's about it. This guy ate a Cessna airplane, it took him two years to do it, he died at the age of 57 from "natural causes" – go figure! Digestability is important. Not everything breaks down to the same degree.

The second factor to consider is **nutrient value**. This is the complexity of fat, protein, carbohydrates, vitamins, minerals, and phytonutrients. All of these. Because we need all of them. When we're eating in the course of the day, we want to think of a time capsule as being a day, not just a single meal. A lot of people have this notion that every single meal has to be a complete meal and you have to combine foods and have everything present. No, it's just during the course of the day. You need the complexity to operate your body. Your body is not going to go into crisis mode because you ate an orange and didn't have any protein to go along with it. You have to realize that it's during the course of a day that you need to take in complete nutrient value.

The third factor, and it's very critical to the health of the digestive tract, is **the presence of fiber**. There are two types of fiber – soluble, which actually dissolves and nourishes the cells of the intestinal tract and keeps them healthy, and insoluble, which gives mass and bulk to the fluid that's in the digestive tract so when water is taken in we actually add mass to the excrement. We need to have both soluble and insoluble fiber. When we have enough fiber in our diet, the research studies show conclusively that we have much lower instances of gastrointestinal diseases like irritable bowel syndrome, Crohn's disease, colitis, and cancer. All of those things are decreased significantly with the presence of fiber in the diet. If you want to read more about that, you can go to Dr. McDougall's website (www.drmcdougall.com). He's done a tremendous amount of research in this area and he's got books and videos and other great stuff.

These are the three most important aspects when to comes to food. We have to look at food in this way and ask what's the digestability, what's the nutrient value, and what's the presence of fiber? We're going to look at food in such a way that we can break it up into a matrix. We're going to break food up into five major categories. You can easily remember these, which is the whole idea. The goal is to increase your diet with foods at the top of the ladder and to decrease the foods that are on the bottom.

Kissed by the sun

The top of the ladder, number one, are all the foods that are kissed directly by the sun. They grow in the sun, they're nourished by the sun, they get energy from the sun – those are the things that are designed for the human body. We're talking about vegetables, whole grains, legumes, fruit and a handful of nuts and seeds. Whole grains include brown rice, oats, millet, barley, quinoa, amaranth, rye, spelt and more. There are a lot of grains – somewhere around 200 different varieties of whole grains. On one list, I counted over 150 different vegetables and over 240 varieties of fruit. One science resource listed over 20,000 species of legumes (beans, peas and lentils)! Such a variety! You want to limit nuts to handful a day. They're really high in fat and for a lot of people they can cause gastrointestinal problems if you have too much.

The foods at the top of the ladder have, by far, the highest concentration of nutrients. They, by far, have the best digestability. They break down the best in our digestive system. They are the most compatible based on our enzymes, based on our physiology, based on the chemistry in our body. They break down the absolute best to the molecular level for transferring to the blood stream. They also have the highest degree of fiber – both soluble and insoluble. You could live completely on these foods and never have a deficiency and never have disease because your body is designed to break these foods down better than any other kind of food.

Starch/ground

The second group of foods are what are called starch foods or ground foods. Some of these are grown underground and includes potatoes, yams, carrots, etc. Or, they are ground up from the first category. By the way the spectrum goes not only vertically but horizontally because you can have ground up foods from the sun. For instance, breads and pastas have a wide variety. You can have whole grain breads and whole grain pastas that are very healthy for you that don't have any processed stuff in it, or you can get the so-called enriched flour, breads and pastas that have basically been stripped and had junk added. There's a spectrum. You can get sprouted whole grain bread or Ezekiel bread at Whole Foods or Trader Joe's. There's a variety of breads that are very healthy that don't have any dairy or sugar that are excellent. You don't want to do a lot of the second category of foods, but they are still healthy for you. Especially if you're active, these foods tend to give you more fuel and break down to glycogen very quickly. In fact, one of the best snacks that you can have if you're hiking is a sweet potato.

Most of the time what you should think about doing is having these foods in a mix with the food from level one. You should have the foods that are kissed by the sun and add some foods from the starch category for any lifestyle. ***Healthy foods*** *from the first two groups will support the health and longevity of the intestinal tract. Everything below these will lead to slower degradation of your intestinal tract and will cost you.*

Adapted

The third category is the food that we as human beings have adapted to over many centuries – meat and dairy. We have adapted to these foods, but we're not designed to eat them. Case in point, we didn't always have fire or tools available, but we still survived as human beings. Think about it, we didn't always have refrigeration available. How likely would it be for you to go out into the pasture, find a bull, wrestle it down to the ground and kill it with your bare hands, rip its flesh open with your bare hands and consume it? The reason we have to cook meat is that if we don't, we get very sick. We also have to pre-digest it because we do not digest it at all if you eat it in the raw. We're not physiologically designed to eat meat. It doesn't break down. We do not have the biochemistry in our intestinal tract to break down the chemical bonds in meat. It will break down a little bit and the rest will putrify as it moves down the intestinal tract. That's why it smells so bad when it gets to the end. Think about it – it's been enclosed in a tube with no air for 24 hours at 98.6 degrees. Not very pleasant. We're not designed for meat. That is any animal, including eggs and fish. For more on the science on this, read The China Study.

The other food in this group is dairy. We're not designed

for dairy consumption either. Here's the logical evidence – of all the species of mammals on the face of the earth, name me one species who routinely nurses from a different species of mammal? I asked this question at the UC Davis School of Veterinary Medicine, one of the top veterinary schools in the world. Want to know what they said? There are none. Name me one species of mammal that nurses in its adult stage of life. Again, you don't see that happening. Think about the logic here. We have the Northern Europeans that actually adapted to dairy during very cold periods of time many centuries ago to survive famine and they actually took milk and turned it into butter and cheese and stored it in cold caves. They would store it in the cave and they'd go in and scrape the mold off because it's an aged food and then consume it. We're not designed to digest that. By the way 75% of the world's population cannot break down lactose sugar after age two.

We hear the hype. "Milk does a body good." "You need dairy so you can build strong bones." "We need to have dairy for calcium so we can prevent osteoporosis." That's the advertising. Here are some facts. The countries that have the highest dairy consumption have the highest rates of osteoporosis. The countries that have the highest rates of dairy consumption have the highest rates of diabetes, type 1 as well. We are now seeing the link from having babies get off of nursing from their mothers and getting on to cow's milk at an early age and that being the co-factor for type 1 diabetes. The reality is that milk does NOT do a body good, it actually does it harm. There's tons of research.

If you read The China Study, you will learn the truth about what we have discovered in relation to meat and dairy. We now know that if we increase animal protein in the diet above a certain small level, we turn on the mechanism to initiate and promote cancer. If we drop the animal protein below a very small level, then we turn off the cancer mechanism. The same is true for heart disease, diabetes, autoimmune disorders and other chronic disorders.

Another aspect to meat and dairy is that these foods cause a much higher acidification of the blood. The calcium that dairy provides is negated by the amount of calcium that is leached from the bones due to the acid state in the blood. The body has to try to buffer this acidification with the calcium in the bones. This is another contributing factor to osteoporosis. The irony is that the dairy industry has duped us to believing that the calcium in milk is necessary to build strong bones, and the reality is that drinking milk actually leads to a net calcium deficit.

The reason you don't hear about the adversities of meat and dairy is money. One of the things I realized when I was in medical school, (of course all of us became members of the American Medical Association) was that 50% of the pages in the journal of the American Medical Association are taken up by pharmaceutical ads. There is an intricacy in the economy – the pharmaceutical industry, the insurance industry, the meat and dairy council, the government, the American

Medical Association, the US Department of Agriculture and the Food and Drug Administration. They're all interwoven. This network supports each other in keeping the economy the way that it is around food. It has to. We're talking trillions of dollars. If this information were to get out on a large scale, it would dramatically impact any aspect of this network, so these industries would take effort to make sure the information would be squashed. In fact, in the state of Colorado it is actually illegal to say anything against the meat industry. It is illegal and you can be imprisoned. There is a very tight network and it has a lot of impact. Don't believe everything you hear, consider the evidence, and go from there.

I'm not saying that you have to be vegetarian or you have to be vegan, I just want you to consider the evidence. Like several other leading scientists, ***I advocate for a predominantly nutrient-dense, whole-foods, plant-based diet.*** Here's what most of us think, "I don't care what he says, I'm going to eat whatever the hell I want." We resist the design. We don't want to pay attention to the design, we want to pay attention to what we want for ourselves and what we like. We listen to that internal conversation and we don't pay attention to the truth. Remember what I said at the very beginning of this journey, that there might be some information that your little monkey will quickly rebel against. Remember, the little monkey is insane!

Embalmed

The fourth category of foods I call embalmed. When I was doing laboratory work, one of the things I would do was to take all of the specimens from surgery and prepare them for examination by the pathologist. I would put each specimen in a container of formaldehyde and over the period of a few hours, human tissue, any organ, becomes very rubbery.

The preservatives that you find in food are added in order to have extended shelf life. Doritos have a shelf life of years. Twinkies can last for decades. You can Google 'list of food preservatives.' These amazing preservatives are filled with chemicals and are "lipophillic" which means "fat loving." They have the same chemical nature as formaldehyde; they actually attach to the fat portion of the cell membrane. They attach there and make the cells and the fat real rubbery. So that cellulite you thought you were getting rid of, think again. Those packaged and preserved foods are loaded with these chemicals. Those diet programs that have packaged, preserved foods like Nutrisystem and Jenny Craig are loaded with preservatives. And they just stay in the body and attach to the fat. They actually preserve the fat, which is a very enticing thought, right?

(An audience member asks if canned vegetables would fall into the 'embalmed' category.) Well, it depends on how they do it. There are some organic, canned soups that you can buy and they are fresh packed with no preservatives in them and those are great. What I'm talking about here is the stuff that is loaded with preservatives that are injected to extend the shelf life beyond imagination. It's all to make money. The longer it's on the shelf the longer people will have a chance to buy it. The foods are pickled, if you will, with the preservatives that they are putting in them. They add BHT and sodium nitrate, which is the same stuff that you can make dynamite from.

Another processed food that you may not think about as processed is oil. Yes, even olive oil. Think about how many olives it takes to make one quart of olive oil – a whole lot. As Dr. Esselstyn writes in How to Prevent and Reverse Heart Disease, you're better off without it. They are 100% fat.

Toxics

The fifth level is the toxic level. These foods have toxic side effects that are going to get you. Number one is refined sugar, number two is deep fried foods (especially with trans fatty acids), number three is sodas, and number four is drugs.

Sugar demonstration - Sugar is the number one culprit.

R: Would you be willing to volunteer? What is your name?

K: Katie

R: Thanks for volunteering. We're going to demonstrate what happens when we ingest sugar. I have two glasses here. I'm going to fill them both about halfway up with water and I'm going to put this packet of sugar in one of them. What I want you to do first is drink the water with no sugar. Let's wait

10 seconds. Put your right arm out and I want you to resist me pushing your arm down as hard as you can. OK, great – you can resist me very well. Now I want you to drink from the other glass with the sugar. Let's wait 10 seconds. I want you to resist me pushing your arm down again. Well, that's interesting. There's no strength there at all.

K: Why is that?

R: Sugar attacks to your system so quickly.

Remember I talked about the sugar levels? The entire amount of sugar that your body needs to have is equivalent to one of these sugar packets. That's how much sugar is in your blood stream and it should be maintained within about 10%. So if you have a packet of sugar, you completely doubled the amount of blood glucose. Your brain immediately perceives it as an emergency and wants to manage it because it's too much. It just confuses the system which then goes into survival mode. Remember, the state that your body is in determines everything. If you're running the crisis software you're going to lose strength in your muscles immediately. It's going to attack your system very, very quickly. So the next time you think about that jelly bean or that piece of cake, remember this. You want to avoid sugar at all costs.

Deep fried foods

We've now got more information about trans fatty acids than every before. I'm very thankful that I've seen this in the last 20 years. It wasn't the case 20 years ago. Recently, New York City placed a ban on the use of trans fats in restaurants. These fats become embalming fluid and promote disease.

I often ask people in my seminar if anyone has ever worked in a fast food restaurant where they made french fries. How often do they change the oil? For many, the response is usually about once a month! Can you imagine? Think about what happens to the oil in your car if it stays in there too long. It gets over heated and becomes sludge. Your engine could actually seize. Well, that's what we do to our bodies when we take in that over-heated old oil. It's pure fat and toxic!

Sodas

The basic thing about sodas is to recognize that they are a salt water solution. Here is the base underlying chemistry of a soda - you can take baking soda and white vinegar, combine them together in a glass of water and get "the volcano," and what you've got left behind is carbonated water, otherwise known as a salt water solution. If you were stranded out in the ocean, would you consider it very wise to start drinking the water from the ocean? Of course not. What would happen if you did? You'd get dehydrated. In fact you could get so seriously dehydrated that it could lead to a particular condition, before you died, called delirium. The brain is 80% water. If you dehydrate the brain it has the most serious complications. Is it any surprise that along with the increase in soda consumption, especially in the last ten years, particularly with our youth, we have the same increase in incidence of ADD, ADHD, and other mental problems? Is there any mystery? Sodas are a major problem. Diet sodas, sparkling water- it's still all the same chemistry.

Alcohol

(An audience member asks about red wine.) I'm going to talk about that next – it falls into the next category because it is a drug. Alcohol is a legal drug, caffeine is a legal drug, nicotine is a legal drug. They all have side effects. Alcohol does kill brain cells, it leads to all kinds of complications, and you know that you never want to drink and drive. Some people will say that there are research studies that show that drinking red wine is helpful and beneficial for you. The total package is what we have to look at. If you're doing everything else right – you're exercising 5-6 days a week and you're eating foods kissed by the sun and you don't have sugar or deep fried foods in your diet, then go ahead and have a glass of wine once in a while if you want. But if you do, focus on the better kinds of wine. The better kinds of wine are the ones without the nitrites or sulfites, which are preservatives, so they are healthier for you. Just make better choices. But don't start drinking a glass of wine every night and delude yourself into thinking that it's going to be a benefit for you. Remember, the research that is presented in the media is done so for one purpose, which is to sell more products.

Caffeine

Remember that caffeine is a drug, and all drugs have side effects. The only drugs they bother to tell you about side effects are the ones they advertise on TV – "complications from using this drug include…" But they don't tell you about the side effects of caffeine with all the coffee commercials. Yet, there are lots of side effects, including cystic breasts, kidney stones, kidney damage, elevated blood pressure, increased risk of stroke and heart attack. As my dad used to say, "how about them apples?"

Nicotine

This is so deadly yet people still smoke. I'll just share this story. When I was taking Organic Chemistry at California Lutheran University, Dr. Wiley gave us this information before conducting a lab experiment. "You can choose to either extract caffeine from tea leaves, or extract nicotine from tobacco leaves. However, I feel I should warn you. If you choose to extract the nicotine from tobacco, once you purify it, the nicotine is a deadly poison. So much as one little drop on your skin will kill you almost instantly." We all chose to extract caffeine.

By the way, keep in mind that caffeine and nicotine have very similar chemical structures. Hmmmm….

This completes the food ladder.

Juicing

Juices are refined from fruits and veggies. The thing is when you drink juice, you speed up the digestive process. It can be a little fast. Fruits have fruit sugar in it, which is fructose, which is different than glucose, or the derivatives of glucose. The difference in fructose is that it's a 5 carbon ring sugar and the other sugars have 6 carbons in the ring, for the molecular structure of sugar. The 5 carbons in the ring and the oxygen in the other place, that particular molecular structure does not require insulin. However, too much of a good thing can still be a problem. If you have too much fructose in the system, it's going to lead to an increase in the blood sugar because it gets converted fairly quickly which can lead to problems too. So you don't want to do too much of it. If you're going to drink a juice, drink 100% whole fruit juice. In fact, make your own and combine it with some vegetables. I make juice for my kids and use apples, carrots, pears, broccoli, and spinach and throw it all together. That way you complex it a little bit so it's not so high in just fructose sugar.

Combining foods

The old way of thinking was combining different components at every single meal. Throw all those ideas out. The old way of thinking was that you had to have a certain portion of protein/meat, a certain portion of fat. Here's the new way to view this. ***You just want to consume, every day, foods from these four groups – vegetables,*** *whole grains, legumes, and fruit. That's what you want. Those are your new four food groups, that's it. Yes, it's a nutrient-dense, whole foods, plant-based diet and this is what works best for the human design.* Here's the chart from the Physicians Committee for Responsible Medicine.

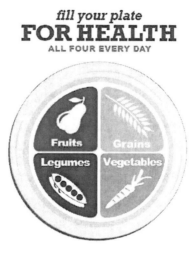

fill your plate
FOR HEALTH
ALL FOUR EVERY DAY

Physicians Committee for Responsible Medicine

Dr. Neil Barnard is a leader and major spokesperson for this group. This is the new food plate. This is what you want to think of in terms of food. You can subsist perfectly fine, I'm living proof and I do not have any protein or any other deficiency. I've been eating this way since 1995.

There are so many more resources online now than ever before, but here are a couple. If you're looking for recipes go to fatfreevegan.com or you can go to veganchef.com and you can get all kinds of recipes and learn how to cook things really healthy. The Engine 2 Diet is a great book. Skinny Bitch has a lot of resources in the back. There are many books to read, cookbooks – there are plenty of resources out there and it doesn't take long to find them. Here's a key – use spices!

The truth about protein

We do need protein. It provides us structure, antibodies, hormones and enzymes for our body that we actually use in a lot of different capacities for all kinds of biochemical functions in our body. There are 20 amino acids that we need in the human alphabet. It's the structure of our body. There are 10 that we need from our diet, the other 10 we manufacture. We only need 10 so it's not like we need whole proteins. It is not necessary to eat whole proteins; that is a myth.

What has happened in our culture is that we came to equate meat with protein. This is not the case. Everything that is alive has amino acids and has the components for protein. All plant matter has the amino acids that we need. They've done the research and shown that soy has 100% of the amino acids that we need for the human body. You do not need to rely on meat or dairy, ever again. It's not necessary.

The truth about cholesterol

When you change your diet, when you change it radically, one of the things that typically happens that most people don't realize is that when you've been ingesting meat you've been ingesting cholesterol. Cholesterol is a steroid. It is the grandmother of the steroid hormones. There are three major derivatives – stress hormones, water regulation hormones, and sex hormones. All of these hormones are derivatives of cholesterol. Cholesterol is the precursor. First we manufacture cholesterol and then we have several biochemical pathways that then break the cholesterol down into these various hormones based on what we need. These are fat-soluble hormones, not water-soluble. They are hormones that stay fairly constant in our body. They get regulated by the pituitary. How many of you have ever been on prednisone or cortisone treatments for anything? When the doctor took you off the medication, did they do so slowly or quickly? Slowly – why is that? There's actually something called a rebound effect. The pituitary is constantly regulating the amount of cholesterol and all of the steroid hormones in your body. When you cut off the supply of cholesterol, your pituitary then has to shift as quickly as possible and then has to compensate for the drop. What happens sometimes when people change their diets and they change it very quickly, the body will then produce more of the hormones, all of the cascading hormones, including things that can agitate you. This is called a "rebound effect." The body goes through a process of re-regulating and it may take a couple weeks or so. It's different for everyone. I've known people who have cut out all meat, dairy, shellfish, and they did it all in one day, and they didn't have any side effects. It's rare, there are usually some side effects. *Most people don't realize that when they're ingesting meat, they're actually ingesting steroids.* It's not unusual to experience some kind of effect from changing your diet. You don't feel well because your brain is having to go through and re-regulate all of those hormones in your body and that takes awhile.

Yes, there is "good" cholesterol and "bad" cholesterol and when you get your cholesterol checked your doctor will measure your HDL and LDL cholesterol. HDL stands for high density lipoprotein and LDL stands for low density lipoprotein. There are actually two other carriers of cholesterol in the body – there's the very low density lipoprotein, and the chylomicrons. You can look all of this up on the internet, there's a lot of good information. The lipoproteins are not cholesterol themselves, they are carriers of cholesterol in the blood. Think of it this way – the HDL is your garbage truck, it picks up the cholesterol and the LDL is your dump truck, it lays the cholesterol down. When your body is out of whack and has too much LDL it has the tendency and predisposition to lay down that plaque. People that have lived with high cholesterol diets have an aorta that feels like peanut brittle because of all that plaque. When your body is in balance you have a lower level of the LDL and a higher level of the HDL and what you want to do is maintain that balance and then what happens is you don't lay down plaque. If your body is acid, and your diet is acidic, you have a tendency to lay down plaque. When the body becomes alkaline you can actually reduce the plaque formation. Many years ago, Nathan Pritikin was a living example of this, and in his subsequent autopsy that he requested, he demonstrated the reversability of heart disease. Dr. Esselstyn's work has verified this as well.

What is the nutritional requirement for cholesterol? How much do you need? Zero. What's the most significant thing that raises cholesterol? Stress on your system is the number one factor that increases cholesterol. Yes, the food that you eat will raise it, but the stress on your system, and running the crisis software will raise it even more. How do we lower cholesterol? Reduce stress and change your diet. Exercise is also another main contributing factor. What's a healthy range for cholesterol? If you actually change your diet significantly, you will actually experience cholesterol levels between 110 and 160. A cholesterol of 200 is not really healthy. The AMA says that because the FDA says that 200 mg per day of cholesterol is your daily allowance for cholesterol in your diet. Insane!

Soy

There's a question that I thought I'd address because it comes up quite a bit. It's about soy. Some people think it's bad for you because it supposedly causes increased estrogen or contributes to cancer while others think it's healthy and the best thing for you. Couple of aspects here...

First, if you read The China Study, we now know that the problem with increasing cancer is not from plant protein, but rather from animal protein. In fact, the research shows that you can have high amounts of plant protein and there is no initiation or promotion of cancer. I happen to feel that it's not the soy that's the problem, but rather the state in which people in – they're surviving. I have not seen any research studies that control for the level of stress in the body.

Another factor is where the soy is coming from. Monsanto has created genetically modified soy and it's called Round-Up-Ready-Soy-Beans. That means that they've genetically altered the soy beans in such a way that the soy plants can be sprayed with Round Up which will kill all the weeds but not the soy. This what most of the soy bean product that is used for feeding the cows, sheep, horses, and pigs – by the way, they've developed corn the same way – and it is toxic. Part of that crop is used to make a lot of your processed foods and they also use it for filler. Now if it's organic soy, that's a totally different story. It doesn't have all of the herbicides and pesticides and this is perfectly healthy.

Research shows that soy, as a single food, has all the essential amino acids that we need for our diet. It matches up perfectly with the human body as far as the amino acid complement. What we've seen is that people who are getting the processed soy foods have some problems that arise. It will raise your estrogen levels if you get the Round-Up-Ready-Soy-Beans. Over 80% of all soy beans grown are Round-Up-Ready-Soy-Beans. I hope that gives you more of an incentive to buy organic. And, if it's stamped as organic from the USDA, don't believe it.

Water

Let's talk a little more about water. Approximately 65% of your body is comprised of water. And it's a fairly narrow percentage. Women typically a little bit more than men. You should be drinking about a half to a full gallon of water per day. Here's a simple test – it's not so much about measuring what you put in, it's consistently drinking enough water that you have consistent output. ***If you are urinating every 1-2 hours, you are taking in enough water. If you are not, consider that you need to take in more water.*** It's really simple.

The best quality water is biodynamically filtered. Usually it's pressed-carbon filtered to take out all of the contaminants, especially the products of chlorination in the water. The other thing is that it should have a high mineral content because that is actually healthy for the health of our heart and for our body as well. I actually buy the water at the Sacramento Natural Foods Co-op. How many of you buy your water? How many of you are spending more than 40 cents a gallon? If you want to spend 40 cents a gallon, go to the Sacramento Natural Foods Co-op, because that's what it costs. You bottle it yourself. It's fabulous water. I've seen it make a difference for a lot of people. The company is called Water Shed and it's actually filtered through the ground and then processed some more. It's biodynamically filtered which means it goes through healthy bacteria in the ground. You bring your own bottles or you can buy bottles there.

Here's your final thing, your hydration tip for the day. Drink a full glass of water in the morning as soon as get up because that hydrates your brain. How many of you drink coffee every morning? You like your coffee? Consider for a moment that your brain does not need the caffeine, it needs the water. If you do this, you'll be surprised, your brain will wake up and will actually function much better.

"To know, and not to use, is not yet to know."

Your mission should you choose to accept it:

1. Stay out of the Red Zone
2. Schedule consistent eating
3. Eat proactively, just enough. It is an experiment.
4. Move up the food ladder.
5. Eliminate the toxics.
6. Drink your water.

I'll close this section with this poem written by Kalidasa in the 4th century in India.

Salutation to the Dawn

Look to this day
For it is life
The very life of life.
In its brief course lie
All the realities and verities of existence:

The bliss of growth,
The splendor of action,
The glory of power.
For yesterday is but a dream
And tomorrow is only a vision,
But today, well lived,
Makes every yesterday a dream of happiness
And every tomorrow a vision of hope.
Look well, therefore, to this day.

CHAPTER 7

SUPPLEMENTATION

The keys to supplementation are very important because this helps you achieve optimum nutritional support. My opinion, and that of many experts today, is that the nutrient value of our soil is not what it used to be 100 years ago. It used to be that we could actually get vitamin B12 from vegetables because they could extract it from the soil. We only have had deficiencies with vegetarians with vitamin B12 because the soil is so depleted. It's not that vitamin B12 does not exist in plant form, it's just no longer available because the soil is no longer rich with organic materials and organic life forms so that vitamin B12 is available to be taken up by the plant. Our lifestyles are different. Few of us have vegetables, farms, acreage, fruit trees and grains in our backyards anymore. We need to supplement because our bodies are not able to get what we need simply from the food that we eat. Even if we get the best quality food, we're still not able to get all that we need. So we need to look at supplementation.

We're going to examine the micronutrients, which are the small nutrients that function like spark plugs for the body. They are important for every biochemical reaction that occurs in your body. We're talking abut thousands upon thousands of reactions that are going on in your body constantly, all day and all night long. All of those have cofactors – particular enzymes that need particular micronutrients to facilitate these reactions. They're going on all the time. For instance, your skin has the ability to stretch. It's called elasticity. That's because you have a particular protein in your body called collagen. Collagen is manufactured all the time. It's manufactured and replaced because we continually use it and break it down. So we need to have our collagen replaced on an on-going basis. You need to have sufficient vitamin C, combined with the amino acid proline, for collagen to function. If you don't have a sufficient amount of vitamin C, you start to lose elasticity in your connective tissue and that means your tendons, your skin, and your ligaments. All of your connective tissue throughout your whole body. One of the direct side effects of nicotine is that it depletes vitamin C rapidly. If you look at a person who has been a smoker for a long time you'll notice one profound thing – they usually have more wrinkles. Most of the time that is the case because they start to deplete the collagen in their skin. That's just to give you an example of how those micronutrients can get involved in the chemical reactions and how they have to be there. We need to have them, and we need to have sufficient amounts of these micronutrients.

There are three major elements that we need to have as micronutrients. The research on vitamins and minerals started back in the early 1900s and a little bit before then. We have books on vitamins and minerals that are really thick. That's based on what we know. There is a lot of information and there is a lot of research going on all the time in terms of vitamins and minerals. They're finding out new things and sometimes it's actually mind boggling how much they're doing. They're trying to figure out the correlation of one specific vitamin or one specific mineral with a particular disease process. My purpose is not to teach you an entire course about all of the individual micronutrients, but rather, how to understand the basics and get what you need.

The first group of micronutrients we're going to discuss are called vitamins. These are compounds that contain carbon in the molecular structure. Some of these are water soluble, like Vitamins B and C. Others are fat soluble, like Vitamins A, D and E. Excess water soluble vitamins can be excreted via the kidneys. However, fat soluble vitamins are not excreted and only break down over time. That is why it is possible to develop a toxicity from too much of the fat soluble vitamins.

The second group of micronutrients are the minerals. These do not contain carbon in their molecular structure.

They have various degrees of water solubility and digestibility based on their chemical structure. For instance, calcium is a needed mineral for the body. If we ingest calcium bicarbonate (chalk), it has a low level of solubility and we get very little calcium. If we ingest calcium citrate (from an orange), it has a high level of solubility.

There is also a classification of micronutrients called phytonutrients. We've been able to study more of these phytonutrients just in the last fifteen-twenty years. Phytonutrients are things that you've probably heard of like beta carotene and lycopene. Those are things that come from plants directly – phyto meaning plant – and there are about 2000 of them. The amount that we need to have in our diet is usually fairly small, and we don't know all the ramifications of phytonutrients and how they interact with our body just yet. The research is just beginning. What is starting to become clear is that you can't have a diet devoid of phytonutrients and still be healthy. It doesn't work. If you had a diet of strictly meat, dairy, and packaged and preserved food, you will not be healthy. You would be devoid of all the phytonutrients. The easiest way to get phytonutrients is to eat real food. Eat the vegetables, legumes, grains and fruit.

How much do we need? The recommended daily allowances, for instance, are pretty arbitrary. It's based on research but the spectrum of the research is huge. They give it their best guess. When you look at the RDAs on food labels, that's called a best guess estimate. What it is for you, nobody really knows.

There is no one gospel truth for how much of any particular micronutrient that you should have. You really don't have to worry abut it if you eat good, quality food, and you get good quality supplements and take them in moderation.

Why should you supplement?

We already talked about the depleted soil. We have poorer quality of food today than ever before. We know this because of how food is processed. Even if it's healthy food, it takes so much more time to get to market. If you don't get organic food, then you'll get food that's been gassed or preserved with something.

Food simply does not have the nutrient value that it used to have. The difference in food that you grow and harvest in your own backyard is so vastly different than the food that you get in the grocery store. Most of us don't have that capability. However, you can get boxes of produce from local organic farmers that have great quality.

We also have busier lifestyles. It's safe to say that we have more stress in our lifestyles than ever before. As a result, our bodies are using and depleting our water-soluble vitamins. All the B vitamins and vitamin C, for example, get depleted much more quickly because of stress. That's another reason to supplement.

It's fairly impossible to get everything that you need just from your food. It used to be said that you could get everything that you needed if you ate really healthy, but today that is no longer the case. Today we have to start thinking about being able to get additional resources to supplement and complement our good, healthy eating habits.

When people are under stress I tell them that they should definitely be supplementing. If they've got a very stressful lifestyle – stressful job, work a lot of hours, sudden changes – that's important to consider, and make sure that you have sufficient supplementation.

Another reason is to prevent or recover from cancer. My mother is a 28+ year survivor of breast cancer. I was in my first year of medical school and that summer I got to go to The Breast Center in Van Nuys. At that time it was the first multidisciplinary approach to addressing breast cancer in the country. It was a novel approach because they had a surgeon, nurse, nutritionist, psychologist – and a whole team of people. One of the things that they stressed was the importance of nutrition and supplementation. My mother made the changes and has been very health conscious ever since. She's been vegetarian ever since and hardly has any dairy at all so she's radically changed her diet. But supplementation has become a part of her life. It's one of the things I've always recommended, and I've had clients faced with cancer, diagnosed with cancer, undergoing cancer treatment and recovering from cancer. Supplementation helps the body to be stronger. We need the antioxidants. We've had more talk about antioxidants in the last few years and that is certainly one part of supplementation.

Another major reason is for sports performance. I know

most of you are not training for the Olympics, but some of you are active. We're seeing more adults choosing to be active than ever before. Just look at how the Boston Marathon has grown! If you're active now and you're planning to be more active, then your body is going to utilize nutrients at a higher rate. So you need to consider supplementation for that purpose as well. As we get older, it's important to understand that we need to support our bodies, especially when it comes to performance or activities.

The final reason is probably the most important reason to supplement - for strengthening of the immune system. If we keep the immune system strong it prevents getting into trouble with diseases, particularly with colds and flu, but with all other major types of diseases as well. Our immune system is not a passive filtration system that you have in an automobile. You have a fuel filter, an oil filter, and an air filter in a car — those are passive filters. They just sit there, they get clogged up, you change them out and put a new one in. We don't have that with our bodies. We have a filtration system but it's active and it's dynamic - like living vacuum cleaners. There are several different components to our immune system. It's got antibodies, lymph nodes, the lymphatic system, white blood cells, the liver, the spleen and more. We've got this entire network that coordinates being able to keep our system clean. So it's really important to have a strong immune system. It requires nutrients for optimum function and a lot of these particular elements of the immune system are very delicate.

Even a small shift or certain deficiency in certain nutrients is enough to undermine the function of the immune system. So we have to make sure we keep it strong.

How do we make sense of supplementation?

Many years ago I was conducting seminars and someone wanted to send me a compendium on supplementation – on all the supplements that were being marketed in the United States - and they wanted my expert opinion on what they should select for their supplementation program. I said I'd look at it so he sends me this book that must have weighed 15 pounds! How do you begin to make sense of it all? One of the things I started to look at was starting to sift through all the hype and marketing. My purpose here is to give you some solid information from which to actually make good choices.

Your first choice of what you should strive to have in your regimen of supplementation are some natural, plant-based supplements. They are basically plants that have been extracted, dried, refined down in a pure form as plants. They are not just extracts of a particular aspect of a plant or a distilled vitamin or a distilled mineral. They are whole-plant material. They are compressed in a tablet/capsule or they're in a powder. There are several companies that have these types of supplements and they're all good. I don't sell any of them, but I've researched them, and I've used many of them. I've looked at their research and development, and in some cases have even gone to their laboratories. I've done most of the homework for you. I'm not the type that just reads the promotional brochure and spends $150. I ask a lot of serious questions, I talk to the scientists and I speak their language.

These are the first choice because they are natural, they are plant-based, and they are not extracts. They are basically portions of real plants. And that's what we need. We need to have a plant-based diet so these supplements are what we need to have in our bodies. And they assimilate perfectly.

The second choice are the pharmacy grade supplements. These are usually fairly expensive and they are distilled or they are chemically manufactured. They are very high quality and usually are manufactured at an FDA approved laboratory. Some pharmacy companies have actually gotten into the business of creating supplements and they sell these at a pretty high price. The problem with these is that they are usually limited because they are just that pure extract of that one, two, or three particular elements. That's all they are. So it doesn't have the complexity and they usually do not have phytonutrients. It's usually a specific vitamin or a specific mineral. For a specific, rare condition where someone actually needs a specific nutrient, these would be warranted.

The third choice is what you see on the shelves everywhere you go. They're generic and you don't know what you're getting. Keep in mind that the supplement industry is not regulated. So you don't know what you're getting unless you do your homework. There are plenty of shenanigans going on out there and it's pretty easy to sell. True story – a particular house in the hills was undergoing some renovations and they decided to take out the septic tank and put in a new one. As they took out the septic tank and started to clean it out, they noticed that at the bottom of the septic tank were all these particular round pills. They realized that they were Centrum vitamins. They never dissolved, they just passed through. There are plenty of things out there that, quite frankly, are covered with shellac.

It is very difficult to test if you have a vitamin or mineral deficiency. So don't fall for people telling you that they can test your hair to find out. The only way to find out is with blood work. And blood work is just one part of it; you'd have to do a lot more than just that. You can test whether or not something will dissolve in your system by putting it in water. If it doesn't dissolve in water, it will not likely dissolve in your system. If somebody approaches you and you are interested, really, really do the research.

Priorities

Your number one priority in terms of your supplementation is that you want to think about strengthening your immune system. This is your foundation for supplementation. You want to keep your immune system strong. You will want to use phytonutrient-rich supplements because those are plant based and that's what is going to help your body stay stronger. A friend of mine wrote a book, he's an MD PhD, he's a brilliant man, Dr. Leonard Ranasinghe. The book is called,

Diet and the Immune System, and he talks about plant-based supplementation to strengthen the immune system.

The second priority is to look at taking a baseline of micronutrients – your basic package of multivitamins and multiminerals. You can take a good comprehensive multivitamin/multimineral. You can get several of those. Whole Foods has a whole bunch of them and Trader Joes has a great one called Super Crusade.

The third priority is to supplement based on any specific needs, whether it's because of cancer, stress or performance, you may need to consider some specific nutrients. For me, I notice that if I take just a little extra calcium and magnesium, it helps prevent leg cramps from when I am playing basketball. You have to figure out what's there for you. This is an experimentation process.

Recommendations

When it comes to plant based supplements, here are a few that I've researched. New ones are coming onto the market all the time. A lot of these you have to order online or get them from a distributor.

One of them is Enerprime. That's the name of the supplement and the company is called Impax. It's very helpful in supporting the immune system. It's all plants. The owners developed that product because their daughter developed alopecia, which is complete loss of hair, when she was eight years old. They went to all the doctors that they could find locally and there was no help for her. They traveled all over the world to see what possible resources were out there. They put together a team of researchers who put together this blend of plants to help reverse the alopecia, and it worked. Then they started noticing that it worked for other ailments with other people. They sent it back out to the lab to see what it was really doing. Alopecia is an autoimmune disorder so they discovered that this particular formula was able to help strengthen the immune system so that the autoimmune reaction stopped. We've known this kind of stuff for years. Harold Hoxie knew this back in the early 1930s because his father, who was a veterinarian, actually taught him how to study the animals and what plants they ate because they could actually reverse their own cancers. They had horses that had a certain skin cancer and all of a sudden they'd start eating certain plants and the skin cancer would disappear. This kind of knowledge and understanding has actually been known in China for over 2000 years. There are other cultures that have known this for centuries, including the Native American culture.

Nutrilite is another company. They have their farms in the San Jacinto valley in Southern California and I've actually been there. They are marketing through the Amway company and they are very good. They've been around abut 100 years. Another one is Juice Plus; it's also very good. They take I think its 17 fruits and vegetables and put it together and it's very healthy. It's an outstanding company with outstanding research and development. Monavie is another one that's come up in the last few years. The big push there is that they've got the corner on the market of the acai berry, which has had a lot of research lately on its health benefits. It's a very healthy fruit. This is just fruit, but it is 19 different kinds of fruits. Nature's Way is a good one that you can get at Whole Foods, Shacklee is another one, Herbalife is another. These companies have done a substantial amount of research and development.

If you get the right kind of supplements combined with a healthy diet, you're going to get all of the things that you need. If you have a crummy diet, all the supplementation in the world isn't going to make a whole lot of difference. It's a waste of money. If you get good supplementation in your body and you do everything else as well, it's a good package deal.

CHAPTER 8

CARDIOVASCULAR EXERCISE

Let's talk about designing the right cardiovascular exercise program for you. Let's have your metabolism go to a whole different level! The major concept that I'm going to present for you is that HOW you exercise is far more important than how much exercise you do. It's not about doing the 'more is better' approach. If twenty minutes on the treadmill is good then forty minutes must be better – no. It's not about how much exercise you do. It's about doing it really well. I know some people who literally exercise two hours a day and wonder why they haven't had any results. So we're going to change things up a bit.

The purpose of cardiovascular exercise is not to burn more calories. It's not to melt away the fat or be in the fat burning zone. You've all seen the machines at the gym that have the fat burning zone on them and people that tell you you're working too hard and you need to be in the fat burning zone. That is hype. Do not go with that. That is not the purpose of cardiovascular exercise. And if you're in that zone, you are most likely under-training. You're not doing it right and you're not doing enough. You've got to be able to be in the right zone. It's not about burning calories or fat.

The true purpose is to build the mitochondria at the cellular level. We're trying to initiate the changes at the cellular level and we want to build more of these mitochondria. The research shows that not only do you build more, but you build bigger mitochondria. The mitochondria take fuel and convert it to energy. The more you build, the more you utilize, and the more energy you produce. We're changing the nature of your engine. We're going from a four cylinder Honda to a twelve cylinder Lamborghini. Every time you exercise from this day forward I want you to remember that you are building more mitochondria. You can start to envision yourself replicating mitochondria. You will burn more fat, all day and all night long, even while you sleep, if you do this right. Would you like to burn fat even while you sleep? That's what we're going to do.

3 levels

There are three major levels of cardiovascular exercise for us as adults. There are actually more, but I don't think anyone here is training for the Olympic trials in swimming so you don't have to worry about any of those other levels. We'll just focus on the major levels. The first two are most important and the third is for those of you who are engaged in any athletic activities and performance.

Number one is what is called the aerobic level. Scientifically, the aerobic level is performed in the presence of oxygen. What we're talking about here, especially when it comes to building more mitochondria, is that there is always oxygen available. What this means, very simply, is that you can breathe comfortably. You've got air. You've got oxygen coming in to your system all of the time and you are not short of breath.

The second level is what is called anaerobic threshold. At this level what we are starting to do is deplete the oxygen somewhat, but not completely. We're starting to get a little short of breath but we can sustain it for a little while. Not for too long, but we'll talk about the parameters and how to set that all up.

The third level is what we call anaerobic. This is where we deplete the oxygen. Your body can still work, amazingly so. For instance, anyone who has done weight training knows what this is like because you work the muscles to the point where they are completely fatigued and sometimes you go past that to the point of failure. You work them to the point that there is no oxygen and they start to hurt. That's working to the anaerobic level. That's not something for everyone, but for those who are interested in performance, it can help. Let's break each one of these down.

Aerobic

The first one is aerobic exercise. I mentioned a little bit about this in a previous chapter, so part of this will be review but it will set the stage for the second level, which is the secret. Aerobic exercise – you must establish complete mastery of this level first. Do not advance to anaerobic threshold training until you have become a master of this level. You must know how to do this. Do not try to go too fast too soon. It will not be to your advantage. Start slowly from where you are and gradually work upwards. Some of you may be at the aerobic level for some time before you start to endeavor to go into the anaerobic threshold level. Some of you may never need to do anything more than the aerobic level. Everybody is different.

Here are the criteria for aerobic exercise:

Number one, to change and alter physiology and start to increase the number of mitochondria, it will require working your way up to 5-6 days a week. Take out your calendars and start to plan to work up to 5-6 days a week. If you have not been doing any cardiovascular exercise, start off at 3 days a week and work your way up. The consistency is really important to establish.

The intensity is also important. This should be vigorous exercise. Start from where you're at. If you're not able to go at a vigorous level now, then you work as vigorously as you can right now. You should work your way until you are able to breathe comfortably, barely. You should not be able to have a long, engaging conversation with the person that you're walking with. That's not vigorous enough. You could talk, but would rather not. Your primary measurement is your exertion so your breathing capacity will tell you everything. If you're breathing comfortably you don't have to worry about your heart rate. That's a secondary measure. If you can breathe comfortably, you're doing great. You're safe.

I want all of you to learn to take your heart rate. You want to check your heart rate for six seconds. You can check it with your radial pulse or your carotid pulse at your neck. You measure your heart rate for six seconds and then multiply the number of beats by ten. You want to check it in the middle of your exercise and particularly at the end of your exercise. Just get in the habit of doing that so you know where it's at, but you're going to rely primarily on the assessment of your breathing. The American College of Sports Medicine talks about what's called the perceived level of exertion, and that's what we're doing with our breathing. There is no ideal heart rate, and you don't have to go by the charts. The charts are statistically based and they are based on a distribution that looks like a bell-shaped curve. We might say that for a particular age group that X is the average so this is where you should be. But in a distribution curve there are some people on either side of the middle. They'll never be in the middle. You'll need to measure your heart rate consistently and determine for you what your particular heart rate is. As you get in better shape, your heart rate will tend to go up higher. You'll be able to put out more exertion and you'll still be comfortable with your breathing. Sally Edwards has a book called Heart Zone Training and she goes strictly by the chart for everybody. As someone who has extensively studied exercise physiology, and having trained hundreds of athletes oever the course of thirty years, I don't agree.

For example, I had a woman in her mid-thirties that came to train with me to run a marathon. She'd run her first marathon and used the training heart rate and she was exactly on target with her training. She ran the first marathon, got to 18 miles and hit the wall. And she'd done everything to the letter. She then came to train with me and had three months to get ready for the marathon in San Diego. Not a whole lot of time to train for 26.2 miles. The first thing I did was test her physiologically. I got her on the treadmill and put a heart rate monitor on her and I started to see where her heart rate would be and yet still be comfortably breathing. Her previous training level according to the charts was 135 to 140. I started her there and kept gradually increasing her intensity and checking to see if she was comfortably breathing and if she could sustain that level of intensity for 20 minutes. 145, 150, 155, 160... Finally, at 165, she was at her maximum aerobic level and still comfortable. Her training heart rate was at 165 for her. That was the level that was still aerobic for her. She was over at the far end of the graph; she was not in the statistical middle. She started training in her true training zone and in three months time when she did the marathon she knocked an hour and a half off her time! That kind of improvement doesn't happen with ordinary training.

You have to know the physiology. When you know the physiology and train physiologically, and you understand what that particular person's individual heart rate zone is for them, then you can train them more effectively.

In terms of duration with regards to aerobic exercise, all you need is twenty minutes at the aerobic intensity. That doesn't include your warm-up or your cool down. How many of you can carve out 30 minutes to make a difference in your energy? Thirty minutes to give you five times more energy in the course of your day? Such a deal!

Exercise modalities

The best types of exercise are the activities that are consistent and keep you moving in a steady state and use as many muscles as possible - recruit as many muscles as you possibly can all at the same time. These are exercises like walking, jogging, swimming, the elliptical trainer, rowing machines, stair climber, and bicycles. Here's a caveat on swimming. You have to know how to swim. Here's the truth – collegiate swimmers have the second lowest body fat of all collegiate athletes, next to the long distance runners. If you know how to swim, are a good swimmer and you know good technique and can sustain it, it can be an excellent exercise.

If you do things that are stop and go, you'd have to do it for a longer period of time. Things like basketball, racquetball or tennis, you'd have to do for a longer period of time to get the same benefits. You get the best benefits from having something that's more sustained when you're at that aerobic level for twenty minutes. What happens physiologically is that you start to stimulate and change the various enzymes and the nature of the messages getting to the nucleus and propagating all the mitochondria. That's what happens over time.

You need to master this level. In collegiate level swimming, we start the season with aerobic training and we do this level of swimming for usually six weeks. We establish the foundation to build the mitochondria. These are well-trained athletes starting the season by working at an aerobic level. You know you've mastered the aerobic level when you are working at your correct heart rate zone and you know when you are there, every single time, without having to read a monitor. You can feel it. Don't rush. Consider that if you're not a well-trained athlete, this will take a while. For most people, I don't push them into the next level for at least 2-3 months, sometimes longer.

Anaerobic Threshold

The next level is the secret weapon level. It is anaerobic threshold. This is the level where it's much more advanced, you've got to have a solid foundation before endeavoring into this and the benefits are amazing. This level can powerfully increase metabolism. The simplest way to describe this is by putting up a little graph.

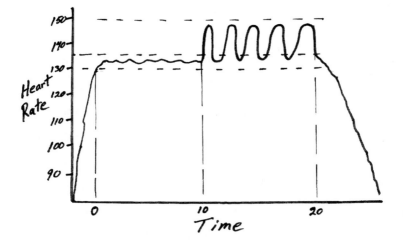

What you want to think about doing is starting off your exercise program and then getting to the aerobic level. The X axis is time and Y axis is heart rate. You've been doing the work and the experimentation for yourself for quite some time. You know exactly where you need to be with your heart rate in terms of your aerobic level. Let's say, for you, that you know between 130 and 135 is your aerobic level. You will start this exercise program with a warm-up and you start the clock as you start to get into the aerobic level. For a normal aerobic exercise session you would stay at this level, get to twenty minutes, and then you would cool down. That would be your aerobic exercise profile. To do anaerobic threshold training what you'll do is the first part exactly the same for the first ten minutes because you need to open up your blood vessels. It's called reaching maximum oxygen perfusion. You need to open up your blood vessels and get the maximum level of oxygen to your muscles. You don't want to start off sprinting or with intervals. That is not safe. After ten minutes you can start to increase the intensity and you're going to increase it about 10%. So this would increase it from about 135 to between about 145 to 150. You're going up to this increased level for a minute and then back to the aerobic level for a minute. You don't go below the aerobic level, you're just going to go back in to the aerobic level. You push it up for a minute to the point where you can breathe barely and you can sustain it for a short period of time. Usually thirty seconds to two minutes is average. For well-trained athletes they can go up to about three minutes of this. You don't want to talk at all. You're breathing fast and you can still manage it and it's consistent. You can do this 1-5 times per week.

It's pretty amazing what happens when you do this. You can change this pattern as time goes on. You can play around with it, and it makes your exercise much more interesting and challenging. You always want to be in control of this when working on an exercise machine. Do not plug in a program on the bicycle or the treadmill that says interval training. You control the intensity. Use the manual program.

A little warning on this – when you are finally ready and you step into doing anaerobic threshold training, you have to be prepared. You may have incredible surges in energy, you may start to drive people in your household crazy because you will be bouncing off the walls and they will wonder what happened to you. This actually happened to one of my clients. She got to this level and a few days later I get a call from her husband and he's wondering what I'm doing to his wife in her workouts because she's up at 2:00 in the morning vacuuming and cleaning! So be prepared, you may have much more energy than you are accustomed to.

What's happening at the physiological level is that you actually get a 10-15% surge in mitochondria. Athletes are used to doing this because this is what they need to do to maximize their performance. This breaks the plateaus. That's another thing that you may notice. If you've reached a level and it's stable and you're doing it well and you've gotten results but they've become stagnant, it's time to kick it up. People sometimes work out for 2 hours at the gym but they can cut their workout time by 75% and have better results.

Anaerobic

The third level is called anaerobic. These are wind sprints. Very advanced and not for just anybody. It can be a powerful complement if you are doing any kind of performance such as basketball or a triathlon, or other activities that involve sprint type action. You need a warm-up before you start doing wind sprints, and you need to be in very, very good physical condition before you can do this. You want to be sure your muscles are strong, you're stretched out, and you should have a physical before you try to engage in this. You can do anaerobic sprints 1-5 times per week, it depends on what your goals are. It's virtually all out. You're pumping your legs and arms as hard as you can. You're not talking at all. You have no interest in talking to anyone. You're working full out. If you're performing, it's great to include this in your workouts. Usually it's a short duration and you get a lot of rest in between. It's really intended to develop those fast-twitch muscles and the capacity for sprinting.

Design YOUR program

You want to start to design your own program. You need to evaluate the reality of where you are right now. If you haven't been engaged in any cardiovascular activity, you start at the base and you start doing it now. Set smart goals. Here's your acronym for SMART – they're Specific goals, they are Measurable, A is for the actions you need to take to accomplish your goal, R is for the resources you need to tap into, and T is for time-frame as to when you want to accomplish this goal. You can set goals in any area of your life using this acronym and you'll be very successful.

Design the action, schedule it, and monitor your progress and your results. Schedule some way of tracking your success and readjust as necessary.

There are different ways to track your cardiovascular fitness. Here are some examples of how you can monitor your progress. One of the things that you can do is check your resting heart rate first thing in the morning, before you even get out of bed. The basic principle is this – as you get in better cardiovascular fitness, your resting heart rate will tend to go down. This means that your heart does not have to work as hard when it's at rest. That's a good thing. Highly trained athletes have resting heart rates in the high 30s to low 40s. The average heart rate is about 72 in this country, but healthy is usually around 60 or less. If you're engaged in this exercise program you'll start to notice some differences.

Another measurement is your performance. What can you do, or what work can you accomplish in a particular distance over time? The formula for work in physics is distance over time. Let's say, for instance, your modality of choice is a stair climber. You measure how many steps you do in those 20 minutes. You start off your program and you are doing 1200 steps. 1200 steps is one step per second. You measure that over time and you set a goal of maybe 2000 steps. You chart your progress and gradually increase and 6 weeks later you are there. Your work performance has improved and you're still breathing comfortably.

Another way is to check your body composition changes. We talked about this in the chapter on fat reduction.

Cardiac recovery rate

This is a simple little test and it never lies. It always works. You do your warm-up and you do your twenty minutes at the aerobic level only, then you check your heart rate to make sure you're at the aerobic level to make sure you're in that range. Normally when you get done you do a cool down and gradually decrease your intensity of exercise. But for the purposes of this test, and you would only do this once every 4-6 weeks, you end and stop completely. Then you check to see what the pattern of your drop in heart rate over the next five minutes is. So you check your heart rate once a minute for the next five minutes. If you're not in good cardiovascular condition, the drop in heart rate is going to be very little. If you're in excellent cardiovascular condition, your drop in heart rate will be very rapid and you'll get down very close to the resting heart rate. Here's the graph of one of my clients.

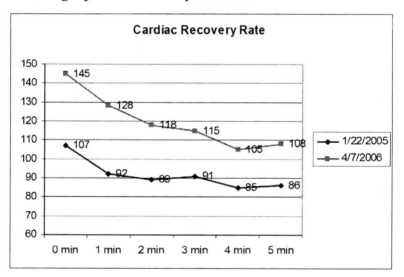

Initially, you would look at him and think he was in shape, but he really wasn't. He wasn't consistent in his cardiovascular exercise. When he first started off, his training heart rate was between 100 and 110. 40 year old man, seemingly healthy, no complications, but he wasn't in cardiovascular shape. His cardiac recovery rate was from 107 and dropped down to 86, he just didn't have a lot of cardiovascular capacity. That was in January of 2005. In April of 2006 I tested him again and his training heart rate was between 140 and 150. He was able to drop down to 108 and he kept going down from there. His cardiovascular capacity had expanded greatly, but since he was not consistent, his recovery rate was not as good as it could have been.

Take out your calendar tonight and schedule your cardiovascular exercise regimen NOW. It will not happen on its own. It cannot be just an idea that sounds nice.

"To know, and not to use, is not yet to know."

Your mission, should you chose to accept it:

1. Stay out of the Red Zone. You do not have the capacity for increasing mitochondria if you get into the Red Zone because you start breaking down muscle protein. You absolutely degrade the mitochondria that you just started to allow yourself to build.
2. Begin to supplement – figure out what you need and start to supplement.
3. Schedule consistency of cardio in your calendar.
4. Determine your modalities, whatever is going to work for you. By the way, it's okay to switch modalities. You don't have to be stuck on one machine for the rest of your life. Do something that you enjoy.
5. Set up your progress measurements, whatever you need to

chart and graph for yourself, do it.

I'll complete this section with a quote that I got from a very dear friend of mine. Many years ago I coached her daughters in swimming and she was one of the first women in the country to ever get a full ride scholarship in swimming. She swam at USC. She loaned me her training log and she actually went to the Olympic trials and she had this quote. I asked her if she wouldn't mind me sharing this with people and she was fine with it.

Value of Training

The duration of an athletic contest is only a few minutes, while the training for it may take weeks, months, or even years of arduous work and continuous exercise of self-effort.

The real value of the sport is not the actual game played in the lime-light of applause, but the hours of dogged determination and self-discipline carried out alone, imposed and supervised by an exacting conscience.

The applause soon dies away, and the prize is left behind, but the character you build up is yours forever.

Don't wait! Start right away!

CHAPTER 9

STRENGTH & FLEXIBILITY

You'll need to dress comfortably for this part since you're going to do some exercises. In this section, you're going to learn how to get rid of aches and pains for the rest of your life! How's that sound?

Here are some interesting statistics. 50% of people over the age of 50 have had a significant bout of chronic back pain. The leading causes of surgery over the age of 60, besides heart disease, are knee replacements, shoulder and hip replacements, and lots of other things like that. We have a lot of orthopedic type problems that happen. Falls are a major concern for the elderly because they don't have core body strength. It is a major, major concern, especially as we get older.

They actually have done research where they have taken people in a convalescent home where 90% of the people in the home were non-ambulatory. That means they were confined to a bed or wheelchair. Only 10% were ambulatory. They started a strength training program for all the non-ambulatory. In two months time, 90% of the convalescent home was ambulatory! The body gets stimulated when you challenge it. ***If you don't use it, you lose it! That's a law of the planet.***

We're going to learn how to challenge the body. Not to be a body builder. I've trained people to do body building. Do you know anyone who has done any body building? Is it easy to be a body builder? No. Does it hurt to be a body builder? It can, and it usually does. If you're going to be successful at it, you're going to have to push yourself really, really hard. How much time would you spend in the gym if you were body building? It's a lot of time. About two hours a day. Anybody got that kind of time? I don't. It's not necessary to go the route of body building.

What we are going to talk about is being able to get stronger. Anybody can do this. And then we're also going to talk about flexibility.

We're going to delve into how we get stronger and how we can do it effectively. We'll contrast body building versus strength training. And we'll also talk about flexibility. We're also going to get a chance to do some exercise. You'll experience some work for yourself. So let's have some fun.

The purpose of this section is to establish the priorities

for strength and flexibility that work with your body's design. It doesn't take a whole lot of time, nor a whole lot of effort. You can do it in just 15 minutes a day. You've got 30 minutes for cardio, 10 minutes for strength, 5 minutes for flexibility – you're done in 45 minutes! I'm going to provide you with a most efficient approach so that you can make positive behavioral changes in your fitness program.

The four basic energies – I want you to consider for a moment that how we are as human beings is that we have an integration of four basic energies - physical, emotional, mental and spiritual. One affects the other, they are integrated. Our physical energy affects our mental energy, our emotional energy, and our spiritual energy. It really does make a difference in terms of how we feel and how our bodies function. Does a stronger body lead to a more spiritual body? Absolutely, yes! Why do you think the Eastern traditions practice martial arts as part of their spiritual practice? They are grounded in spiritual principles and values. It was the monks who had all the secrets of the martial arts. The Shaolin monks in China and Tibet have practiced marital arts for centuries and they know how to take care of their bodies and are incredibly strong. They practice intensely and are very disciplined. We need to have strong physical energy in order to be at our best.

We talked before about the energy model and how the body is like a car and what drives the car is the HeadMaster. Based on your habits that you choose, your HeadMaster chooses the software. Your strength work and flexibility is all reflective of this. It all integrates with what your HeadMaster is going to choose. You don't want to ignore this.

When it comes to the functions of your muscles, what we notice is that protein synthesis is affected by which program you are running. Your body has the capacity to synthesize protein or break it down. We talked before about how when we get into the Red Zone, what happens to protein? It starts to break down. We don't want to see that happen. Now the opposite of breaking down protein is protein synthesis, or, building it up. You can only build protein by running the thriving software. If you're running the crisis/survival software you have limited capacity for protein synthesis. You can't get stronger, you get weaker. You start to break down the muscle protein.

Elasticity starts to break down as well. Elasticity is determined by your collagen and everything in your body's connective tissue. You need to have your body running the happy software because otherwise, in crisis, elasticity decreases. Guess what? You start to get stiffer. You start to get more wrinkles. Stiffness and pain increase.

Have you had back pain? Had any kind of muscle aching pain for some period of time? Consider that back pain and muscle pain are not caused by a deficiency of darvocet, ibuprofen or vicodin! They're not caused by those things. They're generally caused by a deficiency of strength. What generally happens when we go to the doctor, they give us drugs and tell us to go home and rest. That is absolutely the worst thing we can do! What we need to do is challenge the body and make it stronger.

I know for myself, when I start to have pain in my lower back, since I have a scoliosis, I'm being given a message. Strengthen the back! So I start doing my strength exercises immediately and within a very short period of time the pain starts to go away. I don't take any medication for it. There's something missing, there's not something wrong. What's missing is the strength so I start to build the strength back up.

Stiffness and pain increase when we're in survival and the opposite is true when we run the thriving software. Metabolism goes up, protein synthesis goes up, elasticity increases and stiffness and pain decreases. Your body is a machine of building protein all the time – protein molecules are used for building hormones, structures, enzymes - we need protein for a variety of different functions. When we're in crisis we actually diminish our capacity to synthesize new proteins.

Building Strength

Let's talk about building strength. If you have any fear of becoming bulky and a body builder, you don't have to worry about that. We're going to work on getting stronger. Remember my adage – growing old is not for sissies. You can be strong.

I'm a big fan of Jack LaLanne. He died recently at the age of 96. At 95 years of age he could kick your butt. I don't see 60 year olds with the kind of energy he had. I still remember being 5 years old and watching my mother exercise to his television program and her using the black bands with the handles that she used to hang up on the doorknob. Every single one of us can get stronger. And it's a very healthy thing. How old does this body look? What is the physiological age of the body?

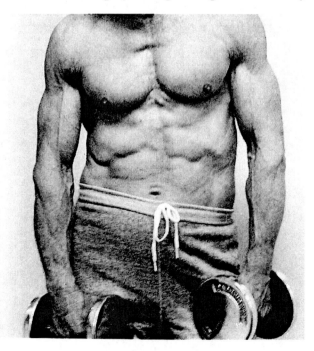

This is not the body of an old man, physiologically. His body is physiologically in the 30s or 40s, yet he's chronologically 67 in this picture. How many 67 year olds have a body like that? He didn't start changing his habits until he was 40. This is the result of consistency 3 days a week. This is John Turner. The picture comes from a book called, Growing Old is Not For Sissies Part 2. The author is Etta Clarke and she had this amazing project of taking pictures of people in their 60s, 70s, 80s, 90s and even somebody who is 100 years old. She took pictures of them in the first book and then 10 years later took pictures of them again to follow up with them. It's pretty extraordinary. These are people mostly in the Bay Area - people who have amazingly, completely altered their lifestyle – quit smoking, quit drinking, took up running, now they've run marathons. If you ever have a lack of motivation and need a shot in the arm, get this book. Everyday just open it up and read a story. One of my favorites is Woody who is 87 years old and surfs with the long boards in Hawaii. At 87 he is pictured there with his 8 year old son! Pretty amazing!

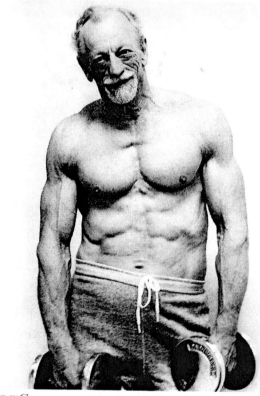

John Turner, age 67

The major concept that we'll address is that HOW you train your muscles and your joints is more important than how much you do. You don't have to do a whole lot. It's about doing a few things really well. It's not about what you train with - what piece of equipment. In fact you can do strength training without any pieces of equipment whatsoever. I'm going to show you how to do extraordinary workouts with just one piece of equipment – stretch bands. You can get them at any sporting goods store.

Benefits of increasing strength.

Number one, it improves your posture. My very good friend, Dr. Eric Wagnon, he's a chiropractor, talks about how he treats people all the time for their spinal alignment and their postural alignment. He works on getting their posture back in balance because that helps the nerves conduct their electricity to the rest of the body which allows the body to function and be healthy. Very important for this to occur, so posture is very important. He does seminars and tells them if they want to maintain their posture, you have to do your exercises and your strength work. Otherwise it's just going to go back out of alignment again and you'll be back for chiropractic adjustments over and over. People often times don't listen and so they come back in and complain about pain and they're just not doing exercises. If you do the exercises, it's quite amazing. If you do the exercises and maintain your posture then your body works, your spinal column is in alignment and the nerves can function because your vertebrae stay in alignment. The only way they're going to stay there is if your muscles are strong. He took an x-ray of me. My hips are level, so it's not the leg length, but I have a scoliosis and it is fairly significant. He told me that most people with this degree of scoliosis have a significant amount of pain. The reason I don't is because I practice yoga, I do all my strength work and I maintain it. I keep it in check and my disc spaces are fine, even though it's got a curve. The strength work is the key. Otherwise, I would have problems.

Strength improves your balance as well. Balance is very important, especially as we get older. It's important to keep your balance because people end up having falls.

It reduces stiffness and pain, we've talked a little bit about that already, but if you're stronger and if you're in alignment, you don't have as much pain.

It improves your capability for activity. How many of you like to hike and be outdoors and be out in the wilderness? Why not do that for the rest of your life? One of my favorite people is a ski instructor up at Kirkwood and he is over 77 years old. He's been instructing for decades.

It builds a leaner, more sculpted body. Would you like a leaner, more sculpted body?

Basic Muscle Physiology

I'm not going to teach you all the biochemistry, but we're just going to do a few basic things here about the way muscles work. If you understand this basic concept, then it makes it easy to visualize what's actually happening inside your body. If we were to look through a high-powered electron microscope and look at a single muscle cell, we would see these sections in the strands of muscle fibers, which are called myofibrils. These sections are called sarcomeres.

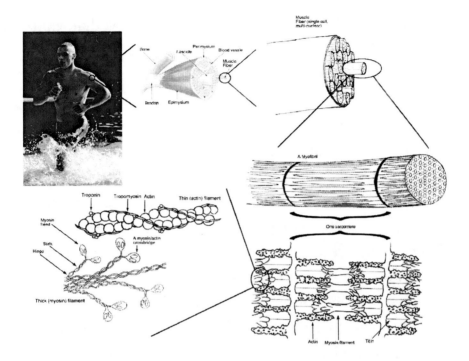

The muscle fibers are very long, the whole length of the muscle. If we're looking at one particular fiber, there are particular sections - sarcomeres. These sections have kind of a wall. In between these sections are some muscle proteins and they have the names myosin and actin. Basically, they slide over each other as we contract our muscles. They have connections at a microscopic level between them, so it basically functions like Velcro. You pull it apart, then press it together and it gets tighter. That's what it's doing, but it's doing it really fast and with no sound effects. It's an amazing design.

There is a law of the planet – if you don't use it, you lose it. It's really simple. If we don't use our muscle, we start to atrophy. The HeadMaster says, "Well, you don't need very much muscle, you're supported completely by that chair, the couch and the bed. You're not doing anything with these muscles. Why do you need them?" What happens over time is you start to atrophy. Do you know anybody who's ever had a broken arm, broken leg, or anything? When you have a fracture and have to wear a cast, your muscles wither. You get out of the cast and you can't move it very easily, it's very stiff. You have to force yourself to start using that muscle again to start to build that muscle back up to where it was before.

When we have a limited number of muscle fibers, we want to be able to build it up. (Volunteer) Give me one finger. I want you to be able hold on to my weight and don't let go of me. It's pretty hard to do that with just one finger. Now give me four fingers and hold on to my weight. He's got more fingers and he's then got more capacity to have more strength. We want to be able to build the muscle fibers. Build more protein cross-linkages and therefore we have a lot more strength and more power to be able to do things. It's interesting that we can actually start to pack it in. We can build a lot more. We can increase this and multiply the number of actin and myosin filaments inside the muscle cells.

With men, you can challenge the muscle and gain a little size depending on how you do your training, your genetics and your testosterone levels. But not necessarily. There are two main types of fibers – fast-twitch fibers and slow-twitch fibers. Men tend to, if they have the fast-twitch fibers and they have the testosterone levels that are high enough, build more girth. However, if we do strength training we don't increase so much in size.

Women don't typically build more girth, however they can build substantially more strength. They just pack it in. So ladies, you don't really have to worry about getting really big.

That's the basis of the physiology. In strength training, muscle protein only builds when the body is challenged. You do not build muscle protein by doing nothing. You can't drink creatine and expect it to happen. A lot of people believe this myth.

Strength training builds bigger pistons. The other thing we talked about in the model was your engine and how many pistons you have in your engine. One of the things that strength training does is help to build more mitochondria, or bigger pistons. That's what we're out to do. A stronger body equals a healthy body, and muscle burns fat all day, all night long. If you have more muscle, you burn more fat. In order for you to have more of these fibers, you have to increase the number of mitochondria because you have to supply more adenosine triphosphate and that's what is used right here at these actin-myosin connections. We use ATP at the muscle connections for strength. If you need more strength, then your body is going to develop more mitochondria. Therefore you use more fuel and you produce more energy. You combine this with cardio and it's amazing what happens.

Strength training versus size training

The most popular things that you'll see in the fitness magazines focus on the concepts that are body building principles. Some of these magazines are getting a little better, and every now and then I see some better articles. But most of the time it's based on body building. Have you ever had a personal trainer? Was it a personal trainer that had a body building background? Most of the time, that used to be the case. How many of you had the trainer that made you do lunges across the floor the first day? Those are body building principles. Building size is only for a few, not very many people really want to do that. Anyone, however, can build strength. And you should.

Principles of body building

The only reason I bring this up is because we're going to contrast this with strength training. I want you to be able to see and distinguish the difference. If you read an article you'll notice the perspective and the philosophy. Here's the body building approach. It's using an approach where you actually train separate body parts. If you ever did body building, you did back and bi's one day, chest and tri's another day, legs and abs another day. Or some formula thereof. That's typically how you do it. You take one section of the body, you blast the living daylights out of it, and then you go home and recover for two days. You break it down so much so your body starts rebuilding while you're resting. You're isolating the muscles and you're attacking them very, very hard to the point, in fact, that it's extreme intensity. It's to the point of failure. You've really done a good job if you're working your biceps to the point where you cannot lift your arms anymore and someone else has to feed you! I actually had a body builder that I used to work out with that got to that point. It's a lot of pain doing it this way and you usually have to rest in between. It's a very different mentality and that's what you usually will read about. They also usually advocate for very high protein, usually high meat, in the diet. I actually knew a guy who went through 16 breasts of chicken every single day. That's a lot of chicken. A lot of people have this notion that in order to build muscle you need a tremendous amount of protein. That's way too much protein. You don't even need close to that amount.

Strength training

I am advocating that you all focus on this approach. This is where we do what are called total body workouts. You work your whole body in one workout. You don't isolate, you utilize what is called multiple muscle recruitment. This is where every single movement incorporates as many muscles as possible in that one movement. It's recruiting as many muscles as you possibly can. This is also about moderate intensity. You only have to go to a level of fatigue, that's it. Your body says you're done and you listen to your body. Do not go to the point of pain, do not cause suffering – just to a point where your body gets tired and if your form starts to break down, you're done.

You may experience some soreness when you initially get started. If you haven't done strength training for a while, you may notice that a little bit. I'm going to encourage you to start off very gradually. You only need to do a little bit. This is not about pushing yourself to get in shape or lose 30 pounds in two weeks and doing everything possible, including spending two hours in the gym every single day. Do not go there. Start off gradually and you may not experience any soreness at all. For these kinds of exercises, you can actually do them every day. As an example - gymnasts and swimmers challenge their bodies every day. Guess what are the two most popular body types that people like to see at the Olympic Games? Gymnasts and swimmers. They are lean, toned, strong, and they challenge their bodies every day. How about dancers? Do they challenge their bodies every day? How many have every seen Mikhail Baryshnikov? What an athlete! He challenged his body every day. Flexible, strong, amazing. You can do these exercises every single day and you just need a healthy, balanced diet.

Priorities

These are the principles of strength training, everybody can follow this.

Number one - here's that word again - consistency. You should start off with at least 3-4 days a week. If you want to change your physiology, you'll work up to doing these exercise 5-6 days a week. And then, once you get to that level, you can maintain your physical strength with about 3-4 days a week.

Start off at 3, ramp up to 6, then when you finally get to the point where you are happy with your strength, you can go back down to 3. I tend to do a little bit every day. Sometimes I skip a day but it's amazing how you can maintain your strength.

Intensity-wise, you only want to go to a level of fatigue. Do not go past that - there is no sense in over doing it. You don't need to get sore, you don't need to get yourself really in trouble, and you don't need to risk injury. That's really critical, especially as we get older.

As for the quality of what you do – everything you do, do it slowly - the slower, the better. Work the slow-twitch fibers in your body. There are different proportions of fast-twitch to slow-twitch fibers for everybody as we're all genetically different. The slow-twitch are the ones that you want to challenge because they help you improve your strength. That's what gives you your endurance, your strength, your capacity to sustain. As for fast-twitch fibers, some people have more than others. The fast-twitch fibers are the ones that tend to grow more in girth. Those are the ones if you wanted to do body building, then I would teach you how to challenge them. It's a very different approach. If you want to be toned, sculpted and strong, slow-twitch fibers are what you want to work on.

The other thing that I'm going to emphasize is that you must maintain spinal stability. As a personal trainer, I would see this as a problem in the gym all the time. You must be very conscientious of the stability of your spine and your posture in every exercise that you do. I cannot even begin to tell you how many times I went into the gym and we'd watch to see how people were doing the exercises, especially in the free weight area and the cable area. We would tally an average of 90% of the people who did not have correct spinal alignment in their exercises. People get injured in the gym very easily because of this. The most common injury in the gym is somebody reaching down to pick up a free weight and they're out of alignment. They don't know how to pick it up. It is critical to maintain spinal alignment.

3 Core Exercises

This is based on research that was done by the National Academy of Sports Medicine, and I was certified by them. Phenomenal work that they do on muscle strength, development and muscle hypertrophy; outstanding training. They had actually done research where they got out EMGs, which is electromyography, and they put these electrodes on all the major muscle groups throughout the body and then had these athletes go through a whole battery of strength training exercises. They fed all of the information into a computer to see what muscles got fired, to what degree they got fired, and then they distilled this information down to see what the fewest number of exercises that we could do that actually fire the maximum number of muscles. They wanted to determine the fewest exercises that incorporate the maximum number of muscles so we could create the most effective workout in the shortest period of time. What they boiled it down to is just three exercises, if we do it right. Three exercises for a total body strength workout! Isn't that great? I've actually been doing this workout myself for 15 years - this is what I focus on. I've trained so many people on them, and my one-on-one clients have actually utilized these in the gym and this is what I focus on teaching them as the foundation. I've had people that want to do body building and a little bit more stuff than just strength, but we always started with this as the foundation and built it up from there. This is always the core group of exercises that I use and teach. Amazing results from doing it this way!

How you do these exercises is what makes the difference. People say "Just tell me the name of the exercises and I can do it from there." No. You can't just know the name of the exercises, you have to know everything about HOW to do the exercise. There are little fine details that can make a huge difference – posture, positioning, form, alignment, breathing, execution, range of motion, range of tension, all of it. A lot of people think they can learn the exercises by just looking at a couple of pictures and that's all they need to do. If you do it sloppy, you're not going to get results.

First thing I'm going to train you on is just posture. Stand comfortably with your feet about shoulder width apart. Focus on the bottom of your ribcage being stretched upward just enough that you feel the stretch in your tummy. Naturally pull your shoulders back. By the way, this is good posture. When you feel that stretch in your tummy, that's good. Notice there's a little tightness is your low back when you do this. That's because your low back isn't strong enough yet. If you sit in a chair for at least a couple of minutes a day, start by sitting in the front of your chair and stretch your ribcage up. You'll improve your posture tremendously. It'll start to make a difference in your alignment and the strength of your core. When we do all of these exercises I want you to feel that stretch. Your abdominal muscles are working, they work all the way around, your low back is working and there are some big muscles in the back and they're working on being able to keep your core nice and strong. When we do all these exercises, keep this core nice and solid and strong by keeping that ribcage up.

Wide-stance squat

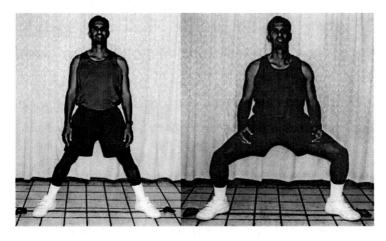

Now, keeping this posture in your torso, move your feet to double shoulder width apart. Gentlemen, turn your toes out 45 degrees, ladies, a little bit more. Bend your knees slightly but keep your core posture. So you're firing your leg muscles just a little bit. If you have serious knee problems, put your hands on a chair in front of you. If you don't have knee problems, you should be fine. By the way, if you do have knee problems, this should make your knee problems better if you do it with support and you do it gradually. You only do this exercise to a point where you feel the muscles being worked. What we want to do here is slowly lower the hips but keep the shoulders back, back straight, keep the core strong. Slowly come down, and come down just as far as you are able to with control. Very slowly come back up. Notice that the hard part is coming back up. Come back up to a point where your knees are slightly bent and your legs are still firing. What we're working on here is called "range of tension" so we're always keeping the muscles firing in this exercise - we never rest completely. Now come down slowly, keep the shoulders back, keep the tummy stretched up, and then slowly come back up. Don't be alarmed at that vibration that is going on, that's perfectly okay. Slowly come down, keep breathing, and then come up nice and slow. Come up to a stand, stretch it out all the way.

To challenge your muscles even more, you can do a few different things. You can come to my yoga class, we do these every time, but we do them a little differently and focus on the breathing. Inhale as we go down, and exhale coming up. Come up to the point where the knees are slightly bent. Now we'll do breath control as we do singles and make life more interesting. Inhale coming down, hold your position, exhale, stay here, inhale, exhale and come up. That gives you a taste of what it's like. We get up to four breaths in my class and you'll build up to it.

You can also add resistance to every exercise you can imagine. You'll see under my feet is a band. You lay it down, step on it, go down and get one handle, get the other, make sure your hips are down, straighten the back, and you come up with resistance. You can also do this with a barbell, with dumbbells, or you can combine. The band is the fastest way to build strength. Progressive resistance is what challenges your muscles most optimally for building strength. In fact, that's the whole concept behind the Nautilus equipment. Nautilus equipment is designed to have an increase of weight and resistance on the muscle at the point where there are more muscle fibers being fired. Genius design.

Row

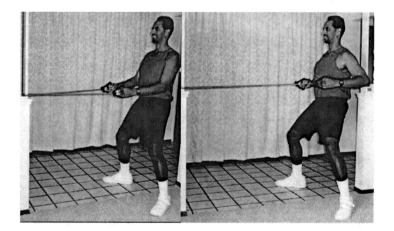

There are different ways to do this. You can do this with cables, you can do this with a machine, you can do it with bands. The key here is to fire the muscles in the rear of your back. There's a big muscle called the latisimus dorsi. It starts down at the base of your spine and goes all the way up to your shoulders - that's the biggest muscle. There's all the other major muscles in the back – we have the trapezius, the rhomboids, the erector spinae muscles - and we want to fire all of them. The most comprehensive exercise for the back, or what we call the posterior muscles, and also for the biceps, is the row.

We're just going to work on the mechanics. Once you get this, then you can do this with any equipment and it'll work for you. Go back to standing with your feet shoulder width apart. Make sure your ribcage is stretched upward, bring the palms up to holding an imaginary tray – so basically your forearms are parallel to the floor and to each other – bring your palms to facing each other and from here what you're going to do is focus on pulling and driving your elbows straight back. You drive them straight back and in the meantime you also pull your shoulders back and open your chest while putting a little extra arch in your low back. Roll your hips back just enough that you feel that arch with just a little extra tightness in that low back. You're tightening everything from the top of your buttocks all the way up to the base of your neck. Now relax and bring your arms forward just a little bit. Notice how just a little movement is enough to relax. Now, we go again. Pull back. Squeeze, you're holding the squeeze now for at least a count of four. Charles Atlas did exercises with just holding the contraction; he didn't use any equipment.

Now, I'm going to show you a modification of this exercise with the band.

There is a way to do the rowing exercise and you use a chair and the bands. What you do is sit on the front edge of the chair and, again, maintain excellent posture. I had horrible posture at one time in my life. I still have to consciously work at it. I have to focus on sitting on the front end of my chair because it gets the core nice and strong. Now, loop the bands around your feet. The wider your stance the more resistance you will have because the bands will be shorter on either end. Cross the bands. Get your shoulders back, ribcage up, and you're going to pull back. You'll tighten all the muscles that we were just working on. Hold it for about four and then slowly come forward.

The part where you slowly come forward is called a negative. This is where you really build your strength - coming forward very, very slowly. Never come all the way out and rest. You want to have a little bit of elbow bend so there's always some challenge to the muscle. What we've found in the research is that the range of tension method builds strength faster than focusing on range of motion. Body building is typically range of motion, strength training uses range of tension. You'll get tired sooner, but that's a good thing.

Notice I'm not breaking my wrists, I keep my wrists straight and am pulling straight back. My spine is perfectly aligned and I'm pulling back nice and slow. This is how you want to do it. If you're not used to it, do it for just a few repetitions at a time.

You can also do this standing up, my favorite is standing up. You can loop the band over the handle of a door. You open a door so that the edge of the door is facing you and you loop it over the door knobs so that the door comes right in the center and then you stand back. That way you've got an equal amount of tubing on each side. You step back, bend your knees a little bit, and now you do the row. (see pictures) Now you're working your legs and your whole core. Everything in your whole body is working very quickly. It's a great exercise - it's one of my favorites. If you can set this up at home, that's your best option.

Chest Press

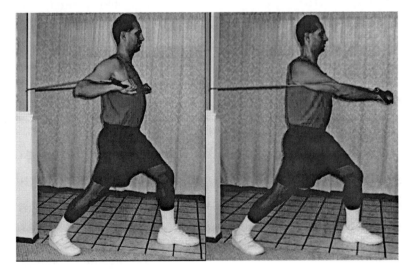

Let's get ready for exercise number three. This will be the chest press. This is going to work all the muscles in the front of the torso. We've worked the legs with the most comprehensive exercise for the entire lower body. We've done the row with the most comprehensive exercise for the posterior of the body. Now we'll do the chest press for all the muscles in the anterior portion of the body, and also your triceps.

Stand back up. Get your feet to shoulder width apart, ribcage is up, bring the forearms up to holding a tray, turn your hands all the way over, and bring your hands into a fist. From here, bring your elbows out 45 degrees from your shoulder. It should be that your hands and forearms are about even with the bottom of the sternum which is called the xiphoid process. Imagine for a moment that your forearms and fists are traveling along a table top at this height. They're not going to go up or down. They'll travel parallel to the floor in a slight arc coming together. Your fists are going to come slightly together but your fists are going to stay on that table top until your hands come together. Then press your fists together and squeeze all the way through your chest. Your elbows are slightly bent and you're really working through your chest. Your ribcage is up, your shoulders are back. Slowly release and bring it back along the table top. Another good practice tool is to do this in front of a mirror so you learn the mechanics. If you're doing it really well you're going to even feel it in your back.

Before I get to the bands, let me show you a couple of the variations. One of my favorite things to do, that is a simple way to do the exercise, is to do an incline pushup against a kitchen countertop. It's a pretty good height for most people. If you're getting started you usually can do an incline pushup against the kitchen countertop. Just take your time. Put your hands on the edge, step back, up on your toes, and get your body nice and straight. You want to get the part of your body where the sternum comes together with the ribs, the 'V' part - you want to get that to come right toward the edge of the countertop. That's your target. As you come down you should be able to come very close to the counter. If you can't come that far down, that's fine. You start by going down as far as you can with control. Eventually you can come down a little bit more. Generally speaking, you can vary the hand placement, don't be uncomfortable, but usually they're a little bit outside of shoulder width. That's where your hands should normally be. You can have them really wide or really narrow if you want to vary things up, but you want to be comfortable. When you come down, you should feel like you've got good control. That's the key. Keep your body very straight, keep your ribcage up, and keep your back straight. Remember your spinal alignment.

The benefit of doing an incline pushup for most people is that you have more control. That's why I teach it this way for most people. A properly done pushup is actually an advanced exercise. I started people who were in their 80s using a dance barre where it was higher but they were using their natural weight to come forward and it was a good place for them to start because they had control and they could do it properly.

Here's a way to do it with the chair, and you can do it with the bands. You sit on the front end, and you hook the bands across the back. You do the same thing – spinal alignment, keep the arms in the right position and this works really well.

If you can, do it like I've got in the picture, standing up. It works everything, your legs, your core.

Training

It takes me 10 minutes to do all of this, at the most. All you need is one set to start off. One set every day. It's not about the number of repetitions, sets, etc. You do it to fatigue and you're done. It's not about how much time you spend, it's the quality of how you do it. The most efficient way to do your exercises is when your body is warm, you want to challenge your muscles when your body is warm, so I do a warm up. Or I do my cardio, cool down and the body is still warm, then I do my strength work, then a little bit of flexibility work, and I'm done. 45 minutes easily, sometimes less. That's what I call the executive workout format. It's very quick, very effective, and it's efficient. You get results. You can challenge your body more intensely as you get stronger. The stretch bands also offer different levels of intensity.

Most people have not been coached on spinal alignment, so without coaching there's a challenge. I see this with all types of gym equipment, they don't give you enough information on spinal alignment. You actually get more results with proper spinal alignment. I used to challenge what I call the 'muscle heads' in the gym because I'm not a big guy, but I'm very strong and I know how to train for strength. They'd look at me and wonder why I was lifting such a small amount of weight. I'd challenge them to use the same weight I was using with exactly my form. I'd have them crying in a matter of a minute and a half. They couldn't handle proper form. It makes a big difference.

Equipment

The best and least expensive equipment, if you want to invest in equipment, is the bands. I really advocate using the bands. They don't cost a whole lot – you can get a good pair for about $15. You can do so many exercises, but you can definitely do your three core exercises with them. You want to focus on using something that is simple and this is portable so if you travel you have no excuse for not exercising. They come in different levels of resistance, different colors, so just find the one that works for you.

Remember that you can use your body weight exercises and you don't need equipment. You can still work your body. You can be in your cubicle at work and still do a strength workout; you don't have to go anywhere.

My other favorite piece of equipment is the exercise ball. It really works your core and you can do so much with it. You can even combine the exercise ball with the bands. Advanced exercises include doing pushups into a ball which will work your core and your upper body unbelievably. Another thing that some people find helpful is to sit on an exercise ball at their desk. If you choose to do that, do it for a little bit of time to start off because your body will rebel if you've not been used to doing that. If you want to build your core muscle strength, trim your waist, and lose some extra weight while you're working, work your way up to just sitting on a ball. You'll be amazed what that will do for you. You'll get much stronger and your back will thank you. Another thing you can do is the squat while holding the exercise ball out in front of you and as you go down, the ball goes up. As you come up the ball comes back in front of you. It's a great exercise. Those are the two of the best. You don't have to go to a gym.

If you do go to a gym and want to use a machine, you need to know how to line your body up properly. Alignment is the key. A lot of machines have seat adjustments and you need to make sure you're seated at the proper height so that you're actually working your muscles at the right level. It's critical; so make sure you set yourself up properly. If you work with a trainer that knows how to set you up, great.

Free weights are actually very advanced pieces of equipment. If you have never trained your body with free weights before, do not think for a moment that you can go out and buy a pair of dumbbells and start working your body and be effective. A lot of people make this mistake. I see women do it all the time. They buy these little 2, 3, or 4 pound dumbbells and I see them with lousy form! I see this in the magazines all the time and they don't talk about posture. Do not go there! You have to really know what you are doing when you work with free weights.

Even more advanced is cables, and this is what the Total Gym is. If you don't know what you're doing as far as body mechanics, you're going to be asking for trouble. You have to know how to control your body. It's a great piece of equipment. And if you know how to work your body and align your body, and you know how to work and stabilize your core, it's great. Chuck Norris knows what he's doing. He's been doing martial arts training nearly all his life. For anything that uses cables, you'll need to be careful. Even the Bowflex is basically a cable machine. It's a good one, but you've got to know what you are doing.

Flexibility

Flexibility goes hand in hand with strength training and it really is the key to longevity. You want to keep your muscles long and you want to consistently do your stretching. It's very beneficial in so many different dimensions.

Some of the benefits of flexibility: improves your posture, it lengthens muscles, it improves your joints' range of motion, it helps you prevent injuries, it reduces stiffness, and it also helps to reduce stress. It's something that you want to practice on a regular and daily basis.

Let's explore some of the principles about how to do flexibility work so you can do it consistently. The basic principles: number one, you need to be in a relaxed state of mind. If you're uptight and tense, it won't work. It's also very good for stress reduction because you just can't stretch when you're uptight. You are best to stretch when your body is warm. However, you can still stretch even when you're cold, you just need to start off very gradually and very slowly. You want to be careful that you don't over-stretch when you're cold because then you have a tendency to injure yourself.

It's best to stretch when you're warm, so the best time is at the end of your workout. I used to work with a couple of gymnasts in helping them improve their flexibility, so we worked on getting them really warmed up first by doing some strength work and getting them stronger with their legs and then doing the flexibility work. You never, ever, ever, ever, EVER want to cause pain. Go to the point of stretch, never to the point of pain.

We're going to work on controlled relaxed breathing. We'll incorporate a very relaxed way of breathing such that you can actually allow your body to very nicely and slowly stretch out more while you exhale. We're going to focus on allowing your body to stretch into the exhale portion of your breath. That's actually when your body can relax the most.

At a physiological level in the muscles, there are these particular little bitty coils - they're called the golgi apparatus. It's basically like a spring, so that the spring holds the limits of how far you can stretch until it knows that you can stretch safely. Generally speaking it takes at least 8 seconds in that particular position before the golgi apparatus start to relax a little bit. They relax only a little bit at a time so you can't go from tension to sudden relaxation, it's gradual. We have this safety apparatus that allows us to stretch a little bit more, but we have to work with it.

Here's some key stretches. There are different areas of the body that you want to stretch – the calves, the hamstrings, the quads, the hips, the abdominals, there's back flexion which is stretching the rear of the back, there's back extension which is stretching the inside of your spine, the shoulders, the arms, and the neck. Those are your major body areas.

There's a great book, aptly titled *Stretching* by Bob Anderson. He goes through stretching very thoroughly, explains stretching, goes through a lot of different routines that you can do for a variety of different sports or different lifestyles. He explains it very well.

Back extension

There is a stretch that is critical for the health of the back. This is back extension. It's the most critical, especially if you've ever had back pain or sciatica. The structure of the spine is such that you have a tin can on top of another tin can, that's your vertebra, and in between you've got a ball of mozzarella cheese, that's your disc. What happens is that if your muscles get weak, then the strapping in between the vertebrae, which is basically like duct tape, that's your ligaments, starts to get weaker and it starts to stretch and get really loose and wiggly.

It starts to compress more on the front end so the disc inside starts to push back. But it pushes back into the spinal canal that has the nerve roots going out and feeding the rest of the body. The disc puts pressure on the nerve, which is what causes the pain because now you've got pressure on the nerve. If you've got constant pressure, that's what is going to cause sciatic pain. In the picture below, protrusion is often referred to as a bulging disc, and it is putting pressure on the nerve root. Prolapse is often referred to as a herniated disc and in this case has completely blocked the nerve root.

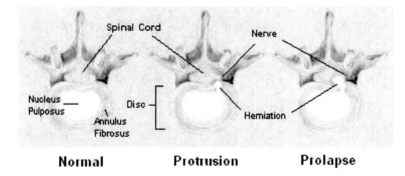

Normal   **Protrusion**   **Prolapse**

What we want to be able to do is take that pressure off by being able to move the discs back into the forward position. We can actually start to manipulate this. Dr. Robin McKenzie in Australia actually created something called the McKenzie Method. It's designed to train people to physically and safely move that disc forward and get the pressure off the spinal cord. This can happen, but you've got to do it properly and gradually. For some people, if they're in back pain, simply lying on a firm surface on their tummy is enough arch of that spine to start to push the disc forward just enough and they'll start to feel it. If you have pain in the moment, you only want to go up to a point where you can tolerate it but it doesn't get to be excruciating pain. You can feel the stretch but it's not painful. It should start to take the pain away. When you do this stretch, you move into as much of an arch as high up as you possibly can. What you'll do is come up from flat with your elbows out and you slowly bring your shoulders up while keeping your hips down and totally relax the back. That will start to take the pressure off the spinal cord. This is Cobra in yoga. It's a critical stretch for the health of your back.

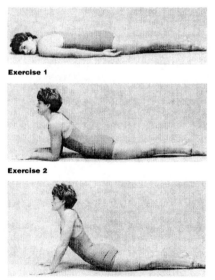

Exercise 1

Exercise 2

Exercise 3

Back flexion

I'm going to show you how to do a forward bend and then we're going to do a little bit of yoga. I'm going to show you a safe way to do what's called a forward bend in yoga, back flexion, or reaching down towards touching your toes. We want to do this safely so you do not injure your back. If you haven't done stretching for some time in your life, you don't want to overdo it. Stand comfortably with your feet a few inches apart and place your palms on your thighs. Use your legs as a support and you're going to slowly bend forwards and have your arms pressing into your legs as you slide your hands only as far down as your knees. Allow your knees to bend a little bit. It is fine to have a little knee bend, in fact, it's preferred. Do not lock out your knees. From here, let your elbows bend and keep your hands on your knees as you support your back and slowly allow your shoulders to come down. Breathe slowly and deeply and just keep your head and shoulders coming down slowly. Once you feel like you're as far down as you can and it feels comfortable, slowly release your hands from your knees and bring your hands down towards your toes. If that is uncomfortable for you, bring your hands back to your knees. Focus on breathing slowly and allow your body to naturally stretch downward a little bit more during the exhale portion of your breath. Relax your head, your neck, your back and slowly let it come down a little bit more with each exhale. To come out of this stretch we'll do it slowly by bringing the hands back to the knees first. Don't lift up, just bring your hands back to your knees only. Slowly straighten your arms, and you can slowly come back up into a stand. This way your back is supported and you won't injure your back. I see a lot of yoga instructors and trainers teaching flexibility work that don't teach you do it properly. If you have your hands on your legs you give your back the support that it needs so you can start to do the flexibility work.

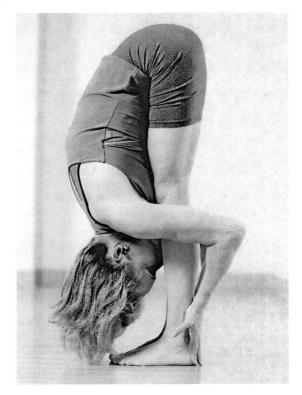

A little yoga

Let's start with a backbend. We're going to bring the hands together with the arms in front and slowly lift the arms up as high as you can, keeping good body posture, and going straight up with the arms. Pay attention to what your body will let you do, but from here slowly arch your low back and bring your head and arms back behind you a little bit. Don't go too far, just go back a little bit at a time. This is also a back extension stretch, but we're doing it standing. Slowly come forward to standing straight and keep your arms up. Take your right hand and grab your left wrist and keep your left arm extended as much as possible and pull your left wrist to the right. This will stretch the whole left side of your body. Let yourself stretch a little bit more with the exhale portion of your breath. Slowly return back to center, switch hands, and pull to your left. Some call this Crescent Moon, some call it Reed pose – depends on which book you read. Relax with the exhale portion of your breath and then slowly come back to center. Take a big, deep breath and release. It feels really, really good.

Design YOUR program

You want to design your strength and flexibility program for you. Each one of you is a unique child of God. Don't copy anyone else, do what works for you. Evaluate your current status. Where are you right now? Where's your strength at right now? What's your flexibility at right now? Design it from where you are at right now. Don't try to force yourself to be anything that you're not. Be honest with your current status. Set some specific, measurable, action related, resourced and time bound goals. That's the SMART acronym that we talked about before. Design your plan of action. You'll need to schedule this. You need to create a schedule for yourself.

Then monitor your progress and results. So whatever you need to do – however many squats you can do holding it for three breaths, design it for yourself. You'll be able to tell what you can do. And then readjust as necessary for you. If you get to a point where you're doing 10 squats and holding it for three long breaths, then ramp it up. Try four breaths per squat and see how many you can do. Challenge yourself a little more, you can readjust. Keep challenging yourself as you need to.

Recommendations

Here are some recommendations on what you can do to get started. One of my favorite recommendations, and of course it's biased because I've been practicing this since I was fifteen years old and I've been teaching this since 1997 - try yoga. I teach my class on Saturday mornings at the Coloma Community Center on 47th and T. It's a wonderful spot. One of the great things about yoga is that you can combine strength and flexibility at the same time. I really like the Yoga Journal's DVDs with Rodney Yee – he's very good. In yoga there are what are called "vinyasas," or routines, where you combine different exercises for a particular purpose. In my class I actually have six different yoga routines. What I find is that having a diversity of these exercises works a lot of different muscles in different ways.

For those of you that are Christian and have spiritual

concerns about yoga, there is actually a form of yoga called Christian Heart Yoga. Remember, it's all good!

You want to develop a strength training routine, whatever works for you. Whether that means you do your core exercises a few days a week or maybe you do yoga a few days a week, make it interesting and challenging and do whatever will work for your schedule.

Practice stretching every day. You can stretch first thing in the morning. You just want to make sure you're doing it very slowly.

Monitor your progress

Here are some things you can look at, you'll notice some changes in your performance so you may have some increases in what you can do. Some body composition changes you'll start to notice – you may get a flatter tummy. You may improve your posture - you may notice that you're standing straighter. You'll actually feel better when you're standing straight. You'll notice flexibility improvements. You'll just want to monitor your progress.

The big thing that I notice for people is that when you start to do this routinely, your chronic aches and pains start to go away. Put this into action. It may be difficult at first, but keep going. Keep challenging your body. It will get stronger and you'll decrease those aches and pains.

"To know and not to use is not yet to know."

Your mission should you choose to accept it:

1. Stay out of the Red Zone. It undermines everything and it's the easiest way we get into trouble. Really work hard at that. I know that people get too busy with their lives and forget to eat or get too busy to eat and fall into the Red Zone.
2. Schedule consistent strength and flexibility exercises for yourself. Create a schedule so it works for you.
3. Determine your modalities – go to the gym, or get some stretch bands or an exercise ball.
4. Set up your progress measurements.

I will close this section with a quote from President Teddy Roosevelt:

"It is not the critic who counts, not the one who points out how the strong man stumbled or where the doer of deeds could have done them better. The credit belongs to the man who's actually in the arena, whose face is marred by dust and sweat and blood; who strives valiantly; who errs and comes up short again and again, who knows the great enthusiasms, the great devotion and spends himself in a worthy cause; who at best knows at the end the triumph of high achievement, and who at the worst, if he fails, at least fails while daring greatly; so that this place shall never be with those cold and timid souls who know neither victory nor defeat."

CHAPTER 10

POWERFUL LIVING

This section will really wrap everything that we've been talking about and pull it together powerfully. I've been teaching stress management since 1987. I started studying stress management when I realized at 2:00 in the morning on a Monday morning before my cardio-patho-physiology exam in medical school that my blood pressure was 170/110. I was sitting down in a chair. 140/90 is considered hypertension and anything above that is definitely high blood pressure. Mind you I could run up and down a basketball court easily for a couple of hours, I had no extra weight, I had no elevated cholesterol and for all intents and purposes I seemed perfectly healthy. But my heart was saying something different. I then got a book that changed my life called *Is it Worth Dying For*, appropriate title, by Dr. Robert Elliott. He's an M.D. and he's one of the leading experts in cardiophysiology - he's a cardiologist. It changed my life because at that point I realized that I was a 'hot reactor'. He had the experience of being a cardiologist and working very, very hard – lots of hours. The first mistake that he came to discover after he had a heart attack was that he didn't listen to his wife who told him to slow down. Second mistake was that he was working too many hours and discovered that he was a 'hot reactor'. He started to discover this whole process on how the body works under stress.

Under short term stress we secrete a hormone called adrenaline. We're supposed to. That's supposed to help us get away from danger. It's what we're designed to do. Remember this whole program is about understanding the design. However, there's another hormone that is secreted when stress is sustained for a long period of time. That hormone is cortisol, which is another one of the steroid hormones. It's one of the derivatives of cholesterol. It starts to get elevated over time and when you have the combination of adrenaline and cortisol what happens is you start to have inflammation and scarring at the blood vessel walls which starts to increase the laying down of plaque. That's what causes the plaque formation. Most recently, studies show that the inflammation can lead to a rupture of this plaque under stress, which then blocks the blood vessel and leads to a heart attack. Be sure to read Dr. Esslestyn's book *How to Prevent and Reverse*

Heart Disease. When you have cortisol being sustained for a long enough period of time it also leads to increased blood pressure because now you're just stressing the body and the system over and over and over again.

I started to realize that I was susceptible to this. My mother has had hypertension, my grandmother and grandfather died of hypertension at a very early age, so I started to realize that genetics were not in my favor. I started studying about stress and reading books about the heart and blood pressure and stress and the psychology about it. I put together this information that I've updated over time.

This was one of the first seminars that I ever delivered. I started conducting this training for nurses at Mercy, Kaiser and Sutter who were in the ICU, the CCU, and oncology and it made a world of difference for them. I did a full eight hour day so this section is a condensation. We did all kinds of things — including deep muscle relaxation, breathing and meditation.

This section, if you embrace it, I promise it will change your life forever. It will make a huge, significant and profound difference in your life. What works for most of us is that we have our systems, our defense mechanisms and strategies and we get triggered and we go to being in survival. This section is about being able to shift that whole process and have peace in your life. We can choose peace and actually have it in our lives. If you've done the *Radical Forgiveness* program, the final step is to choose the power of peace. That's what this section is all about. It ties everything together perfectly.

A little bit of statistics just to give you some information and background relating to stress. In terms of the impact in the workplace, what we see is that healthcare expenditures are nearly 50% greater for workers who report high levels of stress. Who are some of the employees that have high levels of stress these days? State workers, policemen, teachers, firemen – virtually anyone, especially in companies where they are talking about layoffs and potential cut backs. It's no wonder that we have an increase in reported levels of stress in the workplace. It's no mystery. Interesting statistic is that *__the average amount of time off for a stress related incident reported is about 20 days.__* That's a lot of time off of work. I was conducting a seminar for executives down in southern California and one of the CEOs actually mentioned that she had a case where there was an employee that was reporting harassment and stress and she was off for four months and had a pending $150,000 lawsuit. It happens. I was involved at Hewlett Packard; I did my stress management seminar for HP when they were going through their merger with Compaq. There were people off work for at least 6-7 weeks easily. If you talk to doctors that do employee health they'll tell you that problems at work are the major source of stress in workers' lives. It is a major complaint of workers.

The stress is real, but here's what we do – we continue to do the same things over and over again, expecting different results. We prescribe valium, we have people do all kinds of crazy things in response to the stress. Clearly we are suffering from stress and we're not empowered to deal with stress effectively. If we always do what we've always done, we'll always get what we've always gotten. We've got to take responsibility for the fact that we actually cause our own stress. We don't want to think of it that way, but we need to. If we take that position, we can become empowered.

The purpose for this section is to establish the context for how stress actually gets created. How do we create stress and how does it affect us? Once you understand that process, you can do something more effectively with it. Secondly is to identify the three major categories of stress and empower you with very specific strategies to deal with stress effectively in a moment's notice. You'll learn to recognize it and deal with it. Once you have those tools it will make a huge difference. Thirdly is to empower you with a whole new context for creating healthy behaviors. A new framework, if you will, for how you actually deal with the stress in your life. This will make a huge difference.

Let's do a quick review of the energy model from the perspective of stress. The body is just like an energy system and it's just like a plant. We've talked about how all the species of plants are unique and how each species needs their own particular balance of water, soil, light air and nutrients. They all need their own particular, unique balance just like we, as human beings, need our own particular, unique balance. What works for one does not necessarily work for the other. When it comes to managing stress, it's the same thing. For instance, meditation might work for Elizabeth and it might not work for Charlotte. Charlotte may need to dance instead. We have to find out what the balance is for each and every one of us.

When we look at the energy model, stress affects the energy system. When we run the survival/crisis software, it affects the entire system. The whole fuel system gets affected and we then store more food as fat. Our metabolism goes down, our energy goes down, and what happens to the immune system? It gets suppressed. Is it any wonder why we have so many people going to the doctor for colds, flu and allergies when the stress levels go up? You can evaluate the medical statistics and there is such a correlation. The immune system goes down and gets weakened and the mental state becomes depressed. We actually have research studies showing that if we take teenagers who are reporting clinical depression and get them started on an exercise program or out doing things and get them healthy, the depression goes away. When we're in crisis mode, the mental state becomes depressed and when we start running the thriving software it reverses. Let's go to work in figuring out how to do this.

We're going to dive right in to managing stress and figuring out all the skills, tricks and tools that we need. We first need to come to an understanding of how stress really works in our body. *Sometimes what you eat is a little less important than what's eating you.* We have to really look at what's eating you, and I've seen this for many, many people. Stress can be an amazing factor on health, energy, vitality and productivity.

Sources

What are some of the sources of stress in your life? Finances, negative people, keeping medical insurance, time, parents, children, job, imbalance, social expectations, traffic, not having anything to do, too much to do, coping with a health problem, coping with pain, being chastised for being different, death, poor sleep patterns, in-laws, change, politics, divorce, war. Can you relate to any of these sources of stress? These are all the kinds of things that get under our skin. We want to look at the fact that there are many, many kinds of stressors. We're going to take a look at categorizing these soon.

Effects

Let's stop for a moment and consider that these stressors affect us physically, mentally, emotionally, and spiritually. Think for yourself... Of all of the stressors that we were just talking about, what are some of the impacts? There can be depression, high blood pressure, stiff muscles, trouble sleeping, impatience, over eating, trouble focusing, loss of general happiness or peace, you get cranky, difficulty breathing, resignation, sense of hopelessness, feeling limited, loss of appetite, indigestion, digestive problems, alcoholism, addictions of any kind. We know now, more than ever before, that stress combined with a poor diet is the cause of irritable bowel syndrome, Crohn's disease, and ulcerative colitis. It's clearly related. There are many impacts of stress. We now know that 70-80% of all illness has a psychological perspective and component, as well as emotional. We can say that all disease is caused by stress – it's a stress to the system. Our body is in crisis, that is what's happening.

Elements of stress

Now we have to understand how it gets to be this way. We want to look at the basic elements of stress. When I studied this and looked at all of the books that I'd read, I started to realize that everything that we feel as stress is the function of two major things. One, it's a function of what we perceive. We have to first perceive that something is a stressor. That it's a threat or a challenge. If there were a spider on the ceiling in the corner, some of you might perceive it as a threat. Others would simply take a shoe and kill it and that would be the end of it, or maybe wouldn't do anything at all. So it's our perception – that has to be the first element. The second is that we've got to react to it as a stressor. There has to be a corresponding reaction.

In our bodies, for us to experience a stress, we have to first perceive it as such and then react to it as such. If we change one or the other, it no longer has the impact on our body as much as we had before. In fact, this is how we start to train people who have phobias to release their phobias. There's a process called systematic desensitization. Say somebody is really afraid of spiders, we show them a picture of a spider first, really far away. Then they start to be okay with that and we slowly start to bring the picture closer. Then we put an actual spider far away and slowly start to bring it closer so they can actually desensitize.

The reaction to a perceived stressor is an automatic process. We get it over time and condition ourselves. We're no different than Pavlov's dog. Based on everything that's happened in our past, we get to be conditioned and our reactions and perceptions become automatic. It happens without us even thinking about it. It happens at a subconscious level.

One of the things that Collin Tipping talks about is that we think our conscious mind is dictating who we are at any given moment but it only accounts for about 10%. The subconscious is about 60% and the unconscious is about 30%. We think we're being conscious at any given moment, but most of what is running us is our subconscious and our unconscious mind.

We have to realize that is how we're operating and things happen and we react in the blink of an eye and it's not conscious at all. It's automatic. It's been programmed and it's been there for quite some time. What we need to be able to do here is respond as opposed to react. That's what we're going to endeavor to do – look to see how we can respond to it. To do that, we're going to separate stress into three different categories.

These categories are all about levels of control. The first category is what are called external stressors. The external stressors are things that you have very little to no control over. The second category are what is called relationships. In relationships we have some control. We would like to be able to control the other person but have you noticed that we can't? We have control over us, but we don't have control over the other person. Rats! We have some control, but we don't have total control. And the third category are the internal stressors. These are the ones that we manufacture. We create them. We're quite amazing at being able to do this. We have total control.

We're going to spend a little time on each one of these. We've distinguished them, and now we're going to tease them apart and look at what these stressors are like, understand them, and then I'm going to give you some specific tools for each area.

External stressors

Let's start with external stressors. This is the part that you see most of the time in programs that talk about stress management. If you go to any classes on stress management they are going to deal mostly with external stressors. My research has shown that most of the stressors are not in this category so I spend very little time talking about it because where most of the stressors are lie in relationships and internal stressors.

External stressors are the things that you have very little to no control over. Things like taxes, traffic, weather, company policies, foreign policies, federal government, state budgets, state legislators – all kinds of things. You can't do a whole lot about it. You could sign a petition, you could make your phone calls and write your letters, but chances are that you're not going to have that much power to actually make a significant change.

What we need to do here, the strategies - it's about taking care of yourself. The stronger you are the better you can actually cope with everything that is going on. When you're fit mentally and physically you can respond better to circumstances. You have a better capacity to deal with the challenges that come your way. One of the most important things is good nutrition and we've talked extensively about this already – staying out of the Red Zone, eating every 2-3 hours, eating enough to satisfy you. We know that now. Another one is exercise. We talked about cardiovascular exercise, strength and flexibility. All of that is important and we need to practice these as coping skills. Another great strategy is yoga. Another fabulous strategy is meditation. Most people think of the word meditation and think it's really weird, but meditation is really very simple. The real essence of meditation is focusing on one thing such that the chatter in our head starts to be quieted. Massage is a wonderful coping skill. One of my favorite coping skills is partner dancing. You can do non-partner dancing, but for me it's partner dancing. I dance salsa, cha-cha, meringue, bachata, and sometimes tango. It's such an amazing experience because when you're dancing, you have your partner, the music and the dance and everything else floats away completely. I don't care how bad I feel going out dancing, when I leave I'm happy and I have a smile on my face. I feel great.

Controlled breathing

The most powerful coping skill that you can learn to do is controlled breathing, which is actually a form of meditation. We're going to do that right now.

Sit in your chair so that you're relaxed and comfortable. Close your eyes and join me on this little journey. We'll begin by focusing on breathing slowly and deeply as if you're about to go to sleep. Just relax and breathe in through your nose and out through your mouth, relaxing your jaw as you exhale. The next step in this exercise is to now listen to the sound of your breath whispering "ah" with each exhale. You're going to whisper the sound, "ah" quietly to yourself. This is the alpha sound, the first sound of human beings. It is the primary sound that we can make. You'll notice it sounds a lot like the ocean inside a seashell when you place it to your ear. Begin to imagine that you're at the ocean – your favorite stretch of beach, wherever that could be. Just imagine yourself being at the ocean, listening to the sound of the waves rolling gently to the shoreline with each exhale. It is a beautiful, warm, calm, peaceful day. It is perfect, and all is well. Just continue to listen to the sound of the ocean. Relax and enjoy.

I'd love to leave you there but we have more work to do, so when you're ready, open your eyes and come back. I know some of you don't want to leave. What did you notice? Complete relaxation, peaceful, easy, gives you a moment to block out the external. The thoughts will come up, notice them, but don't try to control them. That will drive you even more insane. Just keep focusing on your breathing. Your thoughts will be just like clouds passing by. Don't resist them or try to control them. Just notice them. You can take yourself to a whole different place very quickly.

The studies show that this short little exercise will decrease your heart rate. Practice this consistently and it will bring your heart rate down very, very quickly. It'll also help to lower your blood pressure. In fact, one of the things that I used to train my athletes to do was that same breathing exercise to really get calm and be really focused before their events in swimming. Because when the body is more relaxed, the blood and the oxygenation levels are higher and they actually perform better. It works very well. I started doing this when I was 15 years old and I noticed a difference in my performance in the pool. Everyone thought I was kind of wacky, but I needed every edge possible so I did that and it really made a difference.

Practice doing this every day, and it only takes a couple minutes. If you have a critical decision to make, do this exercise first. I promise you that you will have greater clarity before that decision.

Relationships

Now we're going to delve into the second category of stress – our relationships. Relationships are rather difficult at times, though they can be rather great too.

I want you to think for a moment about somebody that challenges you, even if it's only from time to time. There's a particular challenge that comes up. Write down their name and what you say to yourself about that person in the moment of truth. Be completely honest with yourself. What does that little voice say? This is at the subconscious level and you'd likely never say these things out loud. Things like – you're stupid, you're an idiot, grow up, here we go again, do you even know how to listen? You're not listening to me. How can you do this to me? You make me so mad, get a life, leave me alone... Sound familiar?

Consider that when this little monkey is going off, we are getting upset. We're frustrated and annoyed. We're upset with the other person, the circumstances, the situation, we may even be upset with ourselves. It's normal, it's a natural process, and we all do it. Consider for a moment, if we think about the fact that stress is a matter of what we perceive combined with how we are reacting, does it really have to do with the other person? If it's our perception and our reaction. No, they just happen to be the perfect person to push our buttons – perfectly! If we come from this perspective, then we can have power in the matter. If we are in the position of blaming, shaming and imposing guilt on them, then we have no power in the matter. If we can be responsible and come from 'it's not about them, it's all about me', then if I'm upset, I'm causing it for myself because it's my perception and my reaction. I know it's happening at the subconscious level. I'm not doing this consciously, but I'm doing it. I can be responsible. There are some triggers, some buttons that are getting pushed and God knows this little monkey is going off. That's what is happening. If you come from this perspective, this can empower you.

Self-imposed elements of stress in relationships

Consider there are three primary subconscious conversations of being upset, frustrated, annoyed, irritated, angry and stressed. In the moment of truth when we're upset, one of these three could be occurring.

One is *"I'm not getting what I want."* Do you have children? Remember when they were 2, 3, and 4 years old. Remember what that was like? Consider that when we're upset, we are children in adult bodies. When we're not getting what we want, there is some desire that we have and somebody or something gets in the way! We get upset.

Second is *"This shouldn't be this way."* We create an attachment to how we think things should be. Emphasis on the word "should." You should do this, you should do that, you shouldn't do this, you shouldn't do that, it shouldn't be this way, it should be that way... Our little monkey "shoulds" all over us! Name me the one person on this planet today who is in the position to dictate how life really, truly should be. Is there any one of us on the face of the planet who is in that position? No! Yet, we certainly know people who think they know how life should be and they operate that way. They have an opinion about everything, (have you noticed?) and they must get their way. Consider that we all do this. We get attached to how we think something should be or how it should go. The attachment is the problem. There's a wonderful quote from Dan Millman – ***"Life is not suffering, it's just that you will suffer until you let go of your attachments and just go for the ride."***

Third is ***"Don't say anything. It's not safe. It won't make any difference. Why bother?"*** We consciously suppress saying what is upsetting to us. We stuff it inside and we don't say what we need to say and it just boils, festers and eats away at us inside. We suppress what is frustrating and have all kinds of reasons why we need to suppress it. And WE get stressed in the process. I remember years ago when I was married to my eldest sons' mother and I'd think, "I'm not going to tell her, because if she knows she'll get upset. There's no sense getting her upset so I just won't say anything." Ha! I've since learned that doesn't work. Withholding is actually something that eats away at us.

Look back at that relationship that you wrote down just a few minutes ago and that person that you have an issue with. Of these three elements, look to see which ones are at play in your situation. Is it one, two, three or a combination?

What we need to do to eliminate the impact of getting upset

is to first recognize who is causing your upset. Yes, that would be you. The next step is to realize that it's going to involve communication. The fifth habit of highly effective people (Stephen Covey) is *"seek first to understand, then to be understood."* How we tend to operate as human beings is we say, "I'm going to be understood first before I even begin to think about understanding you. I'm going to get my point across and I'm going to make sure you get it." How's that working for you? That doesn't work. The next thing we'll work on is powerful communication through active listening.

Active listening

We're going to delve into some strategies on how to actually alter relationships by actively listening. It really makes a difference.

We're going to start with active listening. We're going to listen for three aspects. First, the content, which are the words; secondly, we'll listen for the background or the emotion; and thirdly the commitment or the motivation.

Most of us don't listen. Have you ever had a conversation with somebody and they obviously were not listening to you? Have you ever said, "You're not listening to me"? Or maybe you've heard those words. We don't typically listen. What most of us do is this - while I'm hearing the other person talk, I'm listening to my little monkey telling me what I'm going to say the moment he/she shuts up. We think we're listening but we're not. That's the process of the human brain. I actually do a full communication workshop – I've done it for couples and it completely alters the relationship.

We're going to look at these three levels of active listening. The first is content, that's the first thing to listen to. Just listen to the words. Most of us never even have training or practice in doing that. Then we're going to look at the emotion and then the commitment. We're just briefly going to spend some work on this.

Content/words

The first element is to listen to the content.

However, we have to remember our little monkey! Remember that monkey mind I talked about in the beginning? This little monkey is always talking to us, right? No matter what time of the day it is, your little monkey is yaking away! In psychology, we call this your self-talk. And, we're always talking to ourselves. However, with practice, we can learn to displace the self-talk and train ourselves to actually focus on what the other person is saying in the conversation.

We're going to do an exercise and you need a partner for this. This is called a colors exercise. You're going to pick a communicator and a repeater. The communicator's job is to state the names of colors, and please stick with primary colors. And the repeater will say it right after. I'm going to try and move her along as fast as I can. I have to make sure she says it first before I give her the next color. Red, red, blue, blue, green, green, yellow, yellow... You have to concentrate and focus. You have 30 seconds. Ready? Go! Then switch.

Which is easier, being the communicator or being the repeater? The repeater is easier. Why? You don't have to think about what you're going to say. Is it easier to listen or try to get your point across? It's easier to listen, but what we tend to do is spend all this time and energy trying to get our point across. How many of you are involved in work that involves customer service or sales? With this exercise, I just gave you the secret to increasing your sales by at least 20%. When you're being the repeater you are listening to the other person's voice so you are in their world. If you're in sales or customer service, the most important thing you need to be able to do is get into the customer's world. This is a powerful skill. I actually train sales forces in this. Sales go up at least 20%. It's easy. Ever notice that really adept communicators hardly say anything? In fact, Dale Carnegie, who wrote the book *How to Win Friends and Influence People* many, many years ago talked about this process. If you practice really listening and getting what people are saying, you hardly have to say anything and they will call you a great communicator.

Now what we have to do is arrange it so you're sitting next to each other but one of you is facing the screen, the other one is facing the back wall. Here's the exercise. The colors exercise is very simple. You just say one word and repeat it. Life isn't that simple. What we really need to be able to do is listen to what people are saying. We're going to practice the next level - being able to really get when a person states a full sentence.

The person facing the screen will read the sentence when it comes up word for word. Please be sure to read it precisely. After you read the sentence you are then going to listen to your partner attempt to repeat the sentence to you, word for word. There is to be no coaching whatsoever. If they get it correct, you say, "pass". You are done. If they get it incorrect, you say, "no pass". You only get five minutes. Here's the key – this is a partnership. If you're reading the sentence a million miles an hour they're not going to get anything. Be deliberate and be clear. The better you speak it and articulate it so that they can get it, the better they're going to be able to repeat it. This is a team effort because communication is about two people interacting, not just one listening and repeating. This is a team effort. When you're done, switch positions. Count how many times it takes to get to pass.

Here are a couple sample sentences. Practice this exercise with a partner.

> *Tell Peter to put 27 red apples and 34 green pears in the 4 paper sacks and distribute them to the 8 waiting waiters.*

> *Tell Paul to place 31 white flower bouquets and 37 blue place-mats on the 7 tables and unfold 25 of the 43 chairs.*

These exercises were just for content. In the full workshop

I do a lot more work dealing with the emotion and the background and it's extraordinary. I've taken couples through that and it's completely transformed their relationship because they actually started really listening to each other. Can you imagine if the world operated on a level where we really listened to one another? What would the world be like? We wouldn't have the strife that we have, would we? When you're engaged in the partnership of communication, you want your partner to get it and you're committed that they actually get it. And that takes communication to a whole different level other than telling them, "I'm telling you what you need to know, you better get it now and if you don't understand what I'm saying, the hell with you", which is how a lot of people tend to communicate.

I think it's safe to assert that listening is a lot more difficult than we thought it was. I know people that are so good at listening that they can get everything that somebody says immediately. There's also an art to presenting things in such a way that it lands and people actually get it. I coached for 30 years and I know that the communication to my swimmers had to be structured in such a way, deliberately, so that it landed and got translated into action.

Background/emotion

The two other elements in terms of communication, I'll just briefly mention. Next is listening for background. This is where you identify the emotion of what's being said and the feelings that are being communicated. There's a whole list of emotions that we possibly could have in any situation, or that the other person could have. Could be frustration, anger or being annoyed on one end of the spectrum, to being excited, joyful, or anxious in a positive way. There's a whole spectrum of emotions. Gentlemen, we usually don't tend to communicate in such a way where we recognize the emotions of what's being communicated. However, we can be trained. You can start to distinguish and understand emotions. Ladies, you tend to, generally speaking, communicate understanding the emotion and the empathy of the communication much more readily than men do. Men are much more literal, rational, and have a 'get it done' attitude. Women have a lot more emotional expression in their communication. Men, you need to be sensitive to this and understand this, and when you do it really opens the door for communication.

Commitment/motivation

Listen below the words. The deepest level is actively seeking out the commitment. We're always committed to something in any communication, and we have to discover what that person is committed to. Why are they saying what they're saying? We're really getting what's underneath it all. Maybe they're committed to extraordinary customer service. Maybe they're committed to having it go their way. Maybe they're committed to making a difference in peoples' lives. Maybe they're committed to making more money. Whatever the case is, you start to listen to what their commitment is. Not judge them, but listen for it. What's underneath it?

These are the three levels of active listening. In my full workshop I spend more time going through these and we do role-playing and practice.

Internal stressors

Let's delve into the final category and dimension of stress, and that's the internal stressors. These are the ones that arise from inside our own heads. We have total control of them because they are based on our fears. It was perfect in the Sunday service when Reverend Ross talked about FEAR – false evidence appearing real. We make it up inside our own heads. Generally speaking, if we really look, there are some typical fears that stop us. There's something that we say we're committed to yet something gets in the way for us. Our fear gets in the way for us.

Five major fears

These are the five major fears that I've come to look at and study over time that tend to get in the way. The first is the fear of rejection because we have this expectation that we should be able to be accepted. We want to belong and be accepted. We want to be part of the group or part of the social class, whatever the case may be. We hate rejection. How many of you hate being told 'no'? The second is the fear of failure. We all want to succeed. We all want it to work out. We all want it to go well. We have a fear of failure that it's not going to go well. And, we worry that it won't go well. The third is the fear of success. It's a subtle form of the fear of rejection because we become afraid that if we become successful, that we'll have to be more responsible than we want to be, or actually alienate ourselves from the people that we've become comfortable with. For many women that I've coached, they have come to see that they were afraid of losing the weight and becoming responsible for maintaining their boundaries with men. The fat kept them safe and undesirable. I also saw this when I was in medical school because there was a colleague of mine, who is a Latina who had a fear of actually graduating from medical school because if she did, she would completely alienate the rest of her family because they thought that she, being a Latina, should never become a professional. They thought she should get married, have children, and stay at home and take care of her father. There was a fear of becoming a success and being all alone. The fourth fear is the fear of the unknown. We always want to know where we are going and we have a fear of stepping into uncharted territory. We have all kinds of questions and ask all kinds of things before we even step into uncharted territory. We're unwilling to take adventures. The fifth one is the fear of being uncomfortable. If we have a notion or an idea that something is going to be uncomfortable, "I'm not going there." If this is going to be painful or uncomfortable in any way, shape or form, we don't want to do it. It's a real fear for a lot of people. People have their coping mechanisms that they resort to if they feel or they suspect that it's going to be uncomfortable. We stay in our comfort zone.

Think for yourself, when you get stopped, what is the fear that usually is at play there? It could be more than one. Awareness of this will empower you. Remember we talked about creating a breakthrough? You first have to reveal the board. You have to know where the barrier is. If you know what your prevalent fears are, then you can go past them. I know the fear of rejection runs me. I feel I need to be loved. I have a fear of being rejected and not being loved. This stemmed from when I was a baby when I was left in my crib to cry myself to sleep and wasn't held and wasn't told that I was loved. So I have this fear of rejection that got ingrained into my subconscious. It became a very powerful fear. I've since worked through that, and now I recognize that it's just a fear. Sometimes somebody will do something, they'll reject me, and you better believe that it comes up. It's automatic. But now I have some tools to use to help me rewire that pattern in my brain. My fear no longer controls me.

The Four Agreements

The way to conquer fear is to practice living powerfully. Here are some things that are really great. Have you read *The Four Agreements* by Don Miguel Ruiz? It's a wonderful book, one of my favorites. This is one path. There are many paths but it's one of my favorites for living life powerfully.

The first of the four agreements is be impeccable with your

word, second is don't take anything personally, third is don't make assumptions and fourth is always do your best. Let's look at each one of these in a nutshell, and I invite you to read the book.

To **be impeccable with your word** means to speak with integrity. That means no gossip, none whatsoever. No derogatory comments about another person – that's the definition of gossip. We tend to do that as human beings. Speak everything in the direction of truth and love. Not only towards other people, but also to yourself. The hardest agreement is to speak impeccably. Really be honest with yourself. Consistent with this, I remember Reverend Mike Moran said this one time in service and I wrote it down and remembered it ever since – it's an old Arabian proverb. ***"The words of the tongue should have three gatekeepers. First, is it true? Second, is it kind? Third, is it necessary?"*** Before you open your mouth, be sure it qualifies on all three levels. Powerful practice.

The second agreement is **don't take anything personally**. Really, quite frankly, what anyone else thinks of you has nothing to do with you, it has to do with their own drama. It's their own stuff. You don't need to take it personally at all. It has nothing, nothing, nothing to do with you. I love this wonderful quote from a very successful business woman. I heard it about 25 years ago. Somebody asked her what the secret of her success was because she was dynamic, powerful, successful and prosperous. She said, ***"The secret of my*** *success is that whatever somebody else thinks of me, quite frankly, is none of my business."* I realized that there was power in this. She didn't cave in to what anyone else thought of her. That was a powerful demonstration of success.

Third agreement is **don't make assumptions**. When you assume, you know what happens. Find the courage instead to ask questions and express what you really want. Most of us are afraid to communicate and say what we really want. We'd rather withhold. So don't withhold. *Anything can be resolved inside of real communication.* It takes work, and it's not easy. Sometimes the other person doesn't want to play along, and that's okay, still keep at it. It will make a difference.

Fourth agreement is **always do your best**. Do your best at practicing the first three agreements, and do your best at everything else. We're never perfect and sometimes we're tired, sick, or whatever the case may be, but just do your best. Be happy with your best and accept your best.

Powerful love

Don Miguel Ruiz, in his second book, The Mastery of Love, talks about how the opposite of fear is actually love. I'm not talking about emotional or romantic love. I'm talking about powerful love as a practice in one's life - a powerful way of practicing life. In the context of powerful love, which lives inside the domain of thriving, there is no obligation, there is no expectation, it's based on respect. Powerful love is compassionate, always kind and generous, unconditional, and it takes complete and full responsibility.

Five Powerful Practices

This is from an article I wrote. This is where we pull everything that we've talked about together into living an extraordinary and thriving life.

Living inside a thriving lifestyle, we define ourselves from a rare and exceptional point of view. We honor our word, our promises, our agreements and our commitments. We operate from the principles of responsibility, generosity and integrity. We constantly practice the following powerful practices as a way of life.

Acceptance

The first is that of acceptance, this is where we accept others just the way they are with no judgment. This is the basis of powerful love. For anything else is operating from fear. Acceptance is unconditional respect. However, it does not necessarily mean we condone unacceptable behavior. Regardless of the behavior, we accept the person.

Apology

This goes far beyond simply saying "I'm sorry". Apology begins with saying "I'm sorry" but then taking complete responsibility for the impact of your behaviors on others - the ripple effect. Apology includes validating the other person's feelings. The next step is to communicate what you see is missing in both your mindset and your behaviors. Then you complete the apology with a promise and a total commitment to change. "What you can count on me in the future is...." and you fill in the blanks. The practice of apology is therefore ongoing in fulfilling on your promises and commitments. Ladies, would this make a difference if your men could really apologize? I think we know the answer.

Forgiveness

This is where we take any emotional charge about a situation and put it in the past where it belongs, carrying no emotional charge from the past into the present or the future. To forgive, we must completely clean the slate. We recognize that whatever happened, happened. It is done and it doesn't have to shape the present moment or the future any longer. We take complete responsibility for creating our own lives, and therefore, release any resentments towards others. When we forgive others, we free ourselves.

Gratitude

This is where we practice being grateful for what we do have and we stop complaining about what we don't have. What we appreciate appreciates, what we put our attention on expands. A great way to practice this is to declare five things that you are grateful for each day. Another practice is to eliminate all complaining for at least 30 days in a row. If you get to day 29 and complain, start over!

Acknowledgement

This is where we practice communicating to others what we are grateful for about them. We acknowledge their contribution to us and/or others, their actions, and their ways of being. This expands the power of appreciation to others and is a generous gift. When we acknowledge others at every opportunity possible, we initiate a powerful flow of positive energy from us towards others that naturally flows back towards us in many different ways. This is an extraordinary act of generosity that pays huge dividends.

Rest

Some words about rest. You need to get enough rest. Be sure to get what you need. Every single one of us is different. Research studies show that we need to clear out the toxins that we develop during the course of the day - metabolites that we create during all kinds of biochemical processes. Our liver is primarily responsible for cleaning out our immune system, as well as our lymph nodes and our spleen. All of those organs do a lot of the work restoring the health of our body during the course of our sleep. We need to give our livers time to heal and to do their job. The American Sleep Institute did research on people who were overburdened and who were sleep deprived. They put them in a dark room with no stimuli whatsoever and at first they slept thirteen hours, then eleven hours, and they finally regulated out to about eight hours. They kept sleeping at eight hours a night when there was no stimuli, no pressure, and no worries. They balanced out at about eight hours. That's where the research came from that says that you need eight hours of sleep. What they've also since done is shown that if you have a good, healthy exercise program, that can actually compensate for one hour of sleep. Now there's no more excuse to not exercise!

"To know and not to use, is not yet to know."

Your mission should you choose to accept it:

1. Establish consistent self care. Do whatever you need to do to actually be stronger in your body so that you can deal with the stresses that confront you.
2. Practice controlled breathing. It's a wonderful exercise and it will help you to control your stress and deal with the situation at hand.
3. Practice listening. This is a lifelong practice.
4. Practice the four agreements.
5. Practice powerful love.
6. Practice being completely responsible for your life.
7. Practice the five powerful practices.

I close this section with one of my affirmations:

I create my life. I am grateful to have been given the gift of life, and therefore, it is my responsibility to make the most of it, to love more, to live more, to forgive more, to contribute more. I am an extraordinary child of God. I am loving, generous, bold and courageous. Life is an amazing adventure and I am deliriously happy to be living it!

The simple rules:

Rule number one: Don't sweat the small stuff.
Rule number two: It's all small stuff.
Rule number three: Follow rules one and two.

CHAPTER 11

CREATING THE STRUCTURE

This section is where the rubber meets the road. Talk is cheap. Getting lots of information, ideas, going to seminars and getting inspired and motivated – how many of us have done that and two weeks later forgot 99% of it? We're not going to do that at all. This section is about creating a practical, realistic, legitimate structure for putting everything that we've been learning about into practice. Ideas are great, concepts are great, motivation is great, I'm not discounting that whatsoever. But this work is about putting it all into reality, really getting grounded in reality, and having a structure for it to work.

I've coached swimmers for 30 years. I've had athletes swim in college, go to Nationals and even had a couple go to the

Olympic trials. I've had championship teams. Here's what I've noticed over the years. I've had many swimmers come to me and say, "Coach, I want to go to the Olympic Games." What do you think my advice was to them? You've got to come to practice. It's pretty simple. You've got to make it consistently and you've got to be dedicated and you have to be committed and you have to be at practice. You've got to do the work. You have to put it in day after day.

Michael Phelps' coach is Bob Bowman, who I know, and one of my swimmers, Amanda Horrocks, actually swam with Bob and Michael during her college career at Catholic University. And then she came back and swam with me in the summertime and told me, "Coach Ruben I want you to know that you and Bob coach exactly the same way. You have the same mindset, you have the same approach, and you're both focused on the quality and technique. It was so easy to transition from training with you because he has the same approach. Exactly the same." I got to meet Bob in 2002 and we shared a little time and talked, and it's clear that we have the same mindset. Developing champions, like Michael Phelps, is a very systematic approach. In the last two years of his training for the 2008 Olympics, Michael trained seven days a week. Five doubles – five days with double workouts – and two other days of a single workout. Seven days a week. Eight gold medals in the last Olympics. Nobody has ever accomplished that. It's not that he's so much more talented than anybody else, it's that he's so much more consistent than anybody else. That's what it takes.

We're going to take a journey together. We're going to take some time to do some real thinking and create a plan and actually get it ready to set up for yourself. We're going to design the practices. One of the things I did as a coach for years was write out every single workout in advance. I have journals that I collected over years where I wrote down every single workout for every single day. I learned that practice from one of the best coaches ever, Coach John Wooden, who coached the UCLA Bruins to ten national championships. The closest other coach is Mike Krzyzewski at Duke University with four. No other coach has three or more. Wooden demonstrated a level of excellence beyond anybody else. He recorded every single workout. He looked at and he evaluated every year to see what worked and didn't work and how he could fine tune it. I followed his example. I did the same thing for my swimmers year after year. And then I developed a system that worked. It got to a point where I knew the system in my sleep.

I assert that this is what we have to do when it comes to our health. Each of us has to create a system that works. And it's individualized. We have to create a system that works for us and our lifestyle and our practices so that we have a schedule that works, an approach that works, and results that work consistently. I would actually design an entire year of training for my swimmers. I would go to the Board of Directors and give them my plan for the entire year. I had it all mapped out – I had a technical plan, a training plan, mapped out the key competitions three times in the year, the secondary competitions, and what we were going to focus on. I had it all mapped out. 52 weeks planned in advance. Do you think you have a level of success when you have that level of planning? You really do. A lot of my teams rewrote the record books. It's extraordinary when you have a plan.

This section is about developing this kind of a plan. I'm clear this is what we need to do. There are plenty of programs out there where you can learn information about nutrition, but until you have a plan and actually create a new structure for yourself, nothing is going to happen. That's like coming to the swimming coach and saying that you want to get to the Olympics and you have a picture and a vision of it, you see yourself as being an Olympic champion but you never get to the pool. Wishful thinking. We've already established that there is insanity in our culture around us. There's insanity when it comes to trying to create a breakthrough in health, energy and vitality. There are so many programs out there that do the same things over and over again. You can go to Jenny Craig, Nutrisystem, and Weight Watchers, but there's an insanity because it's just not working consistently. It's not enough. We have to take a radical and different approach. "The significant problems we face cannot be solved at the same level of thinking that we were at when we created them."

The purpose of this section is to take a radical approach. Something boldly different. We're not going to do the same things over and over again. We're going to create a breakthrough in relation to time. You're going to have to shift how you actually relate to time and manage your use of time. This will be your breakthrough in time management. You will have benefits not only in your health but in every other area of your life. Would you like to have a breakthrough in how you use your time in your work, in your family, in your relationships and in your health? Multiple benefits just from this section.

We're also going to create a very specific list of goals. Research shows - and Napoleon Hill talked about it for years - that people who declare their goals and just state them have a 1 in 10 chance of being successful. People that write their goals down are about 90% successful. People who have a set of goals written and communicated so that other people hold them accountable are virtually 100% successful. Written goals that are established and communicated and you share it with others holding you accountable – that's what makes a difference. As a business coach and consultant, one of the things that I do is go in to companies and ask them if they have a strategic plan to accomplish their goals. A lot of times they look at me with glass-eyed looks and say no. So then I tell them I should have asked the first question, which is, do you have a written set of goals? If not, that's where we start. I run into business owners and they don't have a written set of goals. They have it just all up in their head. It doesn't work. We're going to create a strategic set of goals. It's a written set of goals with an approach to get from A to Z. It's no mystery. Any organization, any business and any individual who is successful has done the same thing. We're not going to reinvent the wheel, we're just going to use the wheel.

Just to remind you, a breakthrough in performance, a breakthrough in your energy and vitality is going to require three things. All three need to be there. Number one is a shift in mindset, attitude and thinking. That has to occur first. Then, secondly, you have to have a corresponding shift in actions and behaviors. One without the other never works. You shift your mindset but don't change your behaviors, you've got wishful thinking. If you change your behaviors but don't address your mindset, then you're destined to go back to the way it was before. The subconscious will take over. Once you address both of those, you have to get number three in, which is a new structure for support and accountability to sustain the new practices, the new mindset, the way of thinking and the new behaviors. You need to have those in place, otherwise it falls by the wayside.

Here's what I've noticed, and I've learned this from working with many successful coaches – it takes about 21 to 30 days to establish a new habit. Have you heard that before? However, they never gave you the second half of the coin. The flip side of this is that it takes 12-18 months to create a new lifestyle. It takes a lot longer. Rewiring the brain from all the previous conditioning takes time and a structure for success.

Let's talk about creating the structure. What does it take? The major concept here is that failing to plan is planning to fail by default. If you've got no plan, you won't get anywhere. You will most certainly get where you have planned to go – if you've got no plan, you'll get nowhere. If you get on a boat and have no charted course, no destination, where are you going to go? Who knows!?

Assessment

If you turn to the worksheet section, there is a self-assessment form, it's a worksheet. There are two parts to it. The optimum answer for every one of the questions is 10. 10 would be absolutely ideal, perfect, fabulous. Rate yourself – 1 is never, 5-6 is sometimes, and 9-10 is always. Rate yourself from 1 to 10, starting with "I am out of the Red Zone". If you eat every two and a half to three hours perfectly, then it would be a 10. If you're in the Red Zone frequently, if you're in there every day, then you probably would be a 1 or a 2. Somewhere in between, mark it somewhere in between. Take a few minutes now to rate yourself.

There is also a worksheet on body composition. Get your body fat measured and find out what your data is.

The next documents are your goal sheets. This is no different than what a successful business organization will do. They'll create a strategic set of goals. They'll create their goals and then they'll create strategies, milestones, and a tracking system – that's how they'll do it. Every organization that is successful does this. We're going to do the same thing for your health.

Use the self-assessment sheet and body composition sheet as tools to guide you to see what the areas are that you need to work on most. We want to boil it down to no more than 3 major areas. Now, you'll begin to use the goal sheets to write up your goals.

One Minute Goals

The next sheet that you have is about creating one minute goals. It's called One Minute Goals because it takes you a minute, or less, to read it. Once you have worked out your priorities, you want to summarize your goals on these sheets. I actually train my organizations and leaders in being able to use this sheet of paper. Use the acronym of SMART – specific, measurable, actions, resources and timeframe. Do a goal sheet for every single one of your goals. Read it every day, or at least once a week to remind yourself of your goals. I write my goals out every single week. I make sure that I'm fine tuning them and getting more clear about them. It will help you stay focused, which is the key. If you know where your target is, you will get there.

Step one is to be specific and establish a clear goal. What will you accomplish?

Here are some examples of goals:

- Improve my nutrition so that I eat every 3 hrs, eat just enough, and improve my quality to being predominantly plant-based.

- Improve my cardio exercise program to 6 days a week and am fit enough to hike.
- Improve my strength and flexibility such that I eliminate my back pain for good.
- Improve my coping skills such that my blood pressure drops to a normal range and I no longer need medication.
- Improve my relationship skills such that I no longer get upset at work.

Step two is to identify or create the measures. How will you know that you are on target to reach your goal? How will you measure this? What are the indicators? Remember, if you don't measure it, you can't improve it.

Step three is to identify and speculate on the major actions that need to be accomplished towards reaching the goal. What will you do?

Step four is to identify your resources. What resources do you need to tap into, such as people, technologies, information, etc.? Who has been successful at this before? Who can I collaborate with?

Step five is to establish a time frame. By when will you intend to accomplish this goal? Include a timeline for any measures/milestones along the way.

Now it's time to create a NEW structure to implement these goals.

This is a process that we are starting NOW. You don't create a plan, put it on the shelf, let it collect dust and come back to it a year later. This is a dynamic, living, active process. This will take fine tuning and adjusting consistently over time. You'll discover things about yourself and the process. It is ongoing. You want to visit your goals and come back to them over and over again.

Managing Time – Rocks exercise

We're going to talk about managing time and being able to have a breakthrough in time. Do you have challenges in managing your time? Who would like to have a breakthrough in managing time? {Nancy volunteers to help in an exercise.}

What we have here is a collection of rocks of various sizes and we have a bowl full of gravel. Nancy, how are you challenged with your time? What's that like for you?

> **Nancy**: My little voice tells me to get up and do this other thing and I watch the clock go round and round and I allow myself to be late by either being at the computer or reading or doing activities that aren't related to me getting to where I'm going on time.
>
> **Ruben**: Okay, so you're frequently late. Do you have challenges in managing your priorities?
>
> **N**: Yes.
>
> **R**: This is an exercise that's been done for a long time. This jar has all this gravel in it and it's absolutely possible to put all the gravel and all the

rocks in the bowl and have it be below the top. All of it can fit in. I'll give you a minute and a half to solve the problem, with no coaching. You can't force it in.

Nancy struggled with the exercise. First she poured out some of the gravel, then she added some of the rocks, poured in some more gravel, then tried to fit the rest of the rocks in but couldn't. She ran out of time being unable to fit in one of the bigger rocks and some of the gravel.

R: This is a perfect metaphor for how you actually live your life. I'll explain this, and tell me if I'm right or wrong. What you tend to do in how you manage your time is do what is easiest, quickest and fastest to do first. You'll keep doing that until you get all those knocked off until you're confronted by a major priority and you don't have enough time to deal with it. And now you're trying to squeeze it in while squeezing out something else so that you can squeeze that in. Then you're bouncing back and forth between major priorities and you never get all your major priorities attended to. It's quite accurate, isn't it?

N: Yes!

R: It's a reflection of how you live your life. Because, how you do one thing is how you do everything. Now take out all the rocks and all the gravel. This time fill the jar in the order of size with the biggest rocks first, progressing to the smaller rocks, and then put in the gravel.

Nancy was able to fill the jar completely in just under one minute!

In order to get all the rocks in you have to start with the biggest rocks. Get the priorities done first and then move to the smaller stuff. What we tend to do is focus on the minutia. The gravel is the minutia. We do that because it's easy, quick and fast. We tend to go through that laundry list of things because there are a lot of little things and we say we'll schedule time for the big projects but all the little things get in the way and we never get to that big project. What we have to be able to do is get grounded in reality.

Planning sheet

The next thing we're going to do is your planning exercise sheet located in the back. In the left hand column is where you're going to list all of your priorities and all of your major activities. Categorize all the things that are important for you to put time and attention to that you already do right now. Please include sleep, grooming and eating. Include leisure time if that's important to you. You'd be surprised at how many people have no time budgeted for leisure. Once you have your list figured out, in the second column, you are going to list the number of hours that you estimate you are spending in that particular priority or activity per week. For instance, if you sleep 7 hours per day you'll put 49 hours. Once you've got all your activities listed and the hours for each, total up that second column.

Most of us never really take the time to think about what we do with our time. I've done this with business leaders and executives and blown their minds completely. What tends to happen is that we are either grossly over estimating our time or under estimating our time. Most of us are not grounded in the reality of our time. The exact number of hours in a week is 168. No more, no less. If you are grossly under 168, consider that you typically underestimate how you're spending your time. If you're over, you are grossly overestimating how you spend your time. It doesn't matter either way, it's just how we work because we're not grounded in reality sufficiently to know exactly how much time we spend on things.

In the first column, underneath the last priority activity that you listed, now list the things that you would like to accomplish that you have not been engaged in up to this point. Maybe it's strength training, cardiovascular exercise, meditation or cooking differently. There might be some new activities based on the goals that you've created or some new things you need to incorporate into your life. Draw a line under the ones you've been doing up to this point and then write in the ones you need to add in. Then go to the third column, which is the ideal. Without regard for number of hours, what amount of time would do justice for all of these areas that you've identified? What do you feel in your heart would be the appropriate number of hours for all of these areas, including the things you've added in. What would be ideal? Once you have the third column figured out as far as the ideal, then total that column up. It may be 400, it may be 190. Whatever it is, it doesn't matter.

Whatever number you come up with in column number three, the ideal, it now has to be adjusted to become practical so that you can have everything fit under 168 hours. If your number is over 168, you're going to have to do some reduction. This is just like working for a business or (cough, cough) the State of California and making some budget cuts. First you look at the areas that absolutely have to be at a certain level, things that absolutely require a particular number of hours. The other areas, where you can make adjustments, go ahead and make those adjustments. You may have to reduce them by 20%, 30%, or 50%, whatever the case may be.

I also recommend that you create an area on your priorities list for contingency time. You should actually budget in some slack time. Slack time is to be able to deal with life's emergencies as they come up. We all know that life happens and that your plans don't work out exactly as you'd planned. You have to account for that and allocate contingency time. This works in financial management as well. When you actually budget contingency funds, it can really make a difference in your finances. It's no different in how you manage your time. I usually recommend 8-10 hours per week for contingency time. 8 hours is pretty realistic.

This is a process. You'll probably need to go through this exercise several times to get it to work. I do this over and over – usually once a quarter.

Schedule/calendar

Once you create this priority plan, the next step in the process is to create a schedule on a calendar. Use a one week schedule. You're going to start to think about creating a schedule and, like the rocks, you put the biggest priorities in first. You establish those blocks of time first. Allocate them so they are in the schedule. I'm giving you an example spreadsheet in 15 minute blocks of time from 6am-6pm, but you can set it up for 24 hours, your waking hours, or whatever you want to do. Make it reflect what works for you. Create a plan for yourself. Does life always work out so you follow the plan perfectly? No, but you have an idea how to adjust to meet your priorities. It's never perfect, yet it is always perfect. If you have a plan you have an idea of the direction you're going so you can get the big rocks in. That's the key. You don't want to leave getting the big rocks in to the last minute on Friday afternoon. Now you'll just ruin your whole weekend!

	Mon	Tues	Wed	Thu	Fri
6:00am	workout				
6:15					
6:30		breakfast			
6:45					
7:00			shower		
7:15					
7:30				work	

Tracking your goals

Once you've done this, you need to create a tracking sheet for your goals. This is for all your health behaviors. There is an example that is actually from one of my clients. This is what I do. I set people up with a tracking document – we set targeted behaviors and track success every day. It's very simple, yes or no if you did it or not. You track your progress and then you can look to see if you're doing it or not and what areas you need to work on or look to see if there is something missing. This is how you start to assess your progress. If you do not measure, you cannot improve. Edward Demming said that many decades ago and he is the father of quality management.

	Mon	Tues	Wed	Thu	Fri
Out of red zone - eat every 3 hrs or less	y	y	y	y	y
Glass of water upon rising	y	y	y	y	y
No sugar/chocolates	y	y	y	y	y
No starchy snacks	y	y	y	y	n
No beer	y	y	y	y	n

Four Quadrants

You want to be able to focus on using your time wisely. There are four quadrants. This is from Stephen Covey who wrote a wonderful book called *First Things First* - one axis is urgency and the other axis is importance.

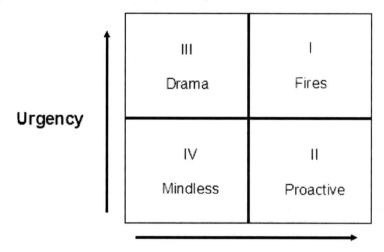

Quadrant number one are the things that are most urgent and most important. They need to be done and they need to be done right now. Basically, they are the fires. Quadrant number two are things that are very important, however, they're not urgent. These are the things that require your proactive mindset and are planned. Quadrant number three are the things that are highly urgent, at least they appear to be, but they're really not that important. Most of the time it is other peoples' drama. Quadrant number four are the things that are not urgent and not important. Those are the things that are mindless. Where you want to spend more time is in quadrant number two, being proactive. If you focus 100% of your time on the 20% that produces 80% of your results, you actually become sixteen times more effective. You want to carve out at least 20% of your time to be in quadrant two. I teach business leaders to work on their business instead of being in their business and carve out 20% of their time so they can actually leverage it and be successful.

What will it take for you to be successful?

1. **Integrity** - making promises to yourself and keeping them. Honoring your word to others and yourself.

2. **Commitment** - dedication to the long term course of ACTION. Never give up!

3. **Being willing to be coachable** - be receptive to others who can contribute to you. Find a coach/mentor to support you and hold you accountable.

"To know and not to use, is not yet to know."

Your mission should you choose to accept it.

1. Continue to evaluate your goals.
2. Continue to revise your plan for how you use your weekly time.
3. Create a daily tracking chart.
4. Increase quadrant two, decrease quadrant one

I'm going share with you one of my favorites.

This is the true joy in life, the being used for a purpose recognized by yourself as a mighty one; the being a force of nature instead of a feverish selfish little clod of ailments and grievances complaining that the world will not devote itself to making you happy.

I am of the opinion that my life belongs to the whole community and as long as I can live, it is my privilege to do for it whatever I can.

I want to be thoroughly used up when I die, for the harder I work, the more I live.

I rejoice in life for its own sake. Life is no "brief candle" to me. It is a sort of splendid torch which I have got hold of for the moment, and I want to make it burn as brightly as possible before handing it on to future generations.

-George Bernard Shaw
Man and Superman

EPILOGUE

In the summer of 2009, I had an amazing spiritual experience. I was on vacation on the big island of Hawaii, and I got to join China Mike on an excursion off the Kona coast – I got to swim in the ocean with the dolphins! A great student of the dolphins, China Mike prepared us by teaching us about the dolphins – how they migrate, what they eat, how they live, and more.

One of the things that struck me was when he told us that the dolphins primarily communicate with each other at a frequency that is at the same level as human emotion. He encouraged us to open our hearts when we were in the water with them and to feel their energy. This is what I did. Fortunately for me, I am an excellent swimmer. I was able to dive down fairly deep and swim alongside them quite a few times – often within just a few feet. Several times, I was eye-to-eye with them, and I just opened my heart with love for them. What I got back was amazing.

"We live in peace. We live in harmony. We live in abundance. We live in love."

What I learned is that we all need to live like the dolphins.

Peace...

Peace is all around us –
In the world and in nature –
And within us –
In our bodies, and our spirits.

Once we learn
To touch this peace,
We will be healed
And transformed.

It is not a matter
Of faith;
It is a matter
Of *practice*.

-   Thich Nhat Hanh

Thank you for giving me this opportunity to share all of this
with you.

Blessings of peace, love, joy, health and happiness,
Namasté
Ruben

WORKSHEETS

SELF ASSESSMENT WORKSHEET

Please rate yourself in each of the following areas.

10 = optimum/always

5/6 = sometimes

1/2 = rarely/never

1. I am out of the "Red Zone......

2. I eat 5-7 times a day......

3. I eat just enough to satisfy every time I eat......

4. I eat 7 servings of "sun" foods a day......

5. I avoid sugar, sodas, fried foods, and drugs......

6. I drink at least 10 glasses of water a day......

7. I take supplements each day......

8. I do cardio exercise at least 5 times a week......

9. I reach maximum aerobic intensity for at least 20 min......

10. I do strength training at least 3 times a week......

11. I do stretching exercises daily......

12. I get 7 to 8 hours of good sleep daily......

13. I am calm, relaxed and peaceful......

14. I take time to take care of myself......

15. I read at least one self-improvement book a month......

16. I have a high level of physical energy all day......

17. I have a high level of positive emotional energy......

18. I am able to focus and concentrate......

19. I am passionate about my work......

20. I feel fully rested when I wake up......

21. I feel positively challenged at work......

22. I view work as an opportunity......

23. I manage my time efficiently......

24. I feel my physical energy stays high every afternoon......

25. I am happy with how my body looks and feels......

26. I enjoy exercise and physical exertion......

27. I am positive and solution-oriented towards problems......

28. I am mentally alert and sharp......

29. I take actions at work consistent with my deepest values......

30. I feel happy and satisfied at work......

31. I get along with my family......

32. I get along with my co-workers/colleagues......

33. I feel organized and mentally prepared to work each day....

34. My personal values are consistent with my actions......

35. I give off positive energy with my voice and body language....

36. I think clearly and logically even under stressful conditions..

37. I feel my work/life is personally fulfilling......

38. I feel sufficiently acknowledged and recognized......

39. I feel confident......

40. I feel fully engaged in the work that I do......

41. I am truly able to leave work behind at the end of the day...

42. My home life does not interfere with my work......

43. My home life restores my energy for work......

44. I feel a sense of purpose in my community......

45. I feel balanced between my work and home life......

BODY COMPOSITION

General body fat percentage categories

	Women	Men
Essential fat	10-12 %	2-5 %
Athletic	13-20 %	6-13 %
Fit - Healthy	21-24 %	14-17 %
Elevated risk	25-31 %	18-25 %
Significant risk	32 % or more	26 % or more

Overweight and obesity raises one's risk of heart disease, hypertension (high blood pressure), stroke, diabetes and cancer. Carrying excess fat stresses the cardiovascular system (200 miles of extra blood vessels for every pound of extra fat) and reduces the body's ability to work efficiently. Additionally, if you have elevated cholesterol and/or blood pressure, your risk increases substantially more.

If your percentage of fat is in the elevated or significant risk categories, you will need to make some lifestyle changes to reduce your risk. Work with a professional to get the support you will need to make lifestyle changes that will stick. Do not delude yourself into thinking you can do it alone!

Body Composition Information

Initial reading

Total weight _____

% Body fat _____

Fat mass _____

Lean mass _____

ONE MINUTE GOAL SHEET

Specific - Clearly establish the goal.

_____

_____

Measurable - What are the measures and milestones that will determine success?

_____

_____

Actions - What are some of the major actions that need to be accomplished towards reaching the goal?

_____

_____

Resources - What resources do you need to tap into? i.e. people, technologies, information, etc.

_____

_____

Time-frame - By when will you accomplish this goal? Include timeline for any milestones.

_____

_____

Follow-up and keeping track

Establish tracking mechanism relative to your goal.

WEEKLY PLANNING WORKSHEET

Activity/Priority	Estimated	Ideal	Plan
Total			

Activity/Priority	Estimated	Ideal	Plan
Total			

RESOURCES

Some good websites for setting up a plant-based diet and much more!

goveg.com

forksoverknives.com

engine2diet.com

fatfreevegan.com

veganchef.com

thekindlife.com

thechinastudy.com

heartattackproof.com

skinnybitch.net

skinnybastard.net

fatsickandnearlydead.com

foodmatters.com

takepart/foodinc.com

calpirg.org

OPPORTUNITY

You have a choice – to survive or thrive – to be ordinary or extraordinary. My invitation to you is to be extraordinary. Repeat after me, "I am extraordinary!" Here's an extraordinary opportunity for you – one on one fitness coaching with me. How it works is that I set up an initial consultation with you that takes about 45 minutes to an hour and a half and we thoroughly go through your medical and fitness background. I help establish your goals and key behaviors that are important to you, I set up a tracking spreadsheet customized for you, and we have weekly calls of about 15-30 minutes where I coach you and provide guidance and support. I'm the biggest cheerleader you can possibly imagine. We all need the support of knowing that we're doing the right things and doing them well. When you know you have somebody in your corner holding you accountable, you get to create miracles. When you are trying to do it on your own and you've got nobody in your corner, nobody cheering you on, and nobody holding you accountable, you will go back to the way it was before, I promise you. That's the reality. I have a 100% success rate with my clients. I don't know of any other program that can claim that. I do. Every single one of my clients does fabulously well. It's an opportunity. You get to choose.

From Healthy Lifestyle Coaching client
Reverend Charles Cooper,
music director, producer, song writer:

Before I started working with Coach Ruben in April of 2010, my life was in a dark, numb, decaying place. I was in a lot of pain both physically and emotionally. I'm 50 years old, 5 foot 7 inches tall, and was at my heaviest weight of 290 (Wow! When I see that number it still freaks me out). My suit size was 52, and my waist was 48. My eating habits were fast food, sodas all day, candy, potato chips, sweet juices, cookies, and of course a real dependency on CHEESE CAKE!

Coach Ruben had gently approached me many times before, but I was not ready to hear his message. I had failed so many times in the past that I thought there was no hope for me. I thank the Universe that Ruben was patient and persistent. He knew that when the student is ready the teacher will show up! I guess you could say I was in the perfect storm of pain. I had just lost my wonderful mother, my health was declining and I had basically given up. My back was up against the wall. My choices were to live or die. I chose to LIVE!!!!!!

Some of the key lessons and insights that I have gotten from working with Coach Ruben include: It's not my fault!!!!!! And, it's never too late to change! In the past I used starvation to diet. But Coach Ruben taught me how to eat, what to eat, and when to eat. He taught me how to exercise and achieve a balance. And all this was done with core spiritual principles.

Since I started working with Coach Ruben, my whole lifestyle has changed! Before I was in a victim state of mind - now my consciousness is rooted in being victorious!!!! I now exercise 6 days a week, which consists of strength/resistance training and cardio. Additionally, I've learned and I continue to learn what to eat and how to eat!

As a result, in just 14 months, I have physically lost over 80 pounds!!! My suit size is now a 42, and my waist is 36. The side effect of losing this much weight is that I look and feel really, really good! I still have a ways to go for me, but emotionally, I have an entirely new level of confidence and direction in my life. Mentally, I have amazing clarity. Spiritually I have a deep abiding sense of peace and purpose like never before.

My advice to those considering working with Coach Ruben: Coach Ruben is a healthy lifestyle coach, with emphasis on LIFE, because through his guidance my entire LIFE has been transformed!

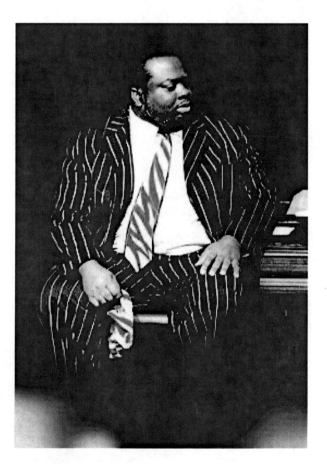

Reverend Charles Cooper - January, 2010
Before working with Coach Ruben
Turn page to see the After photo

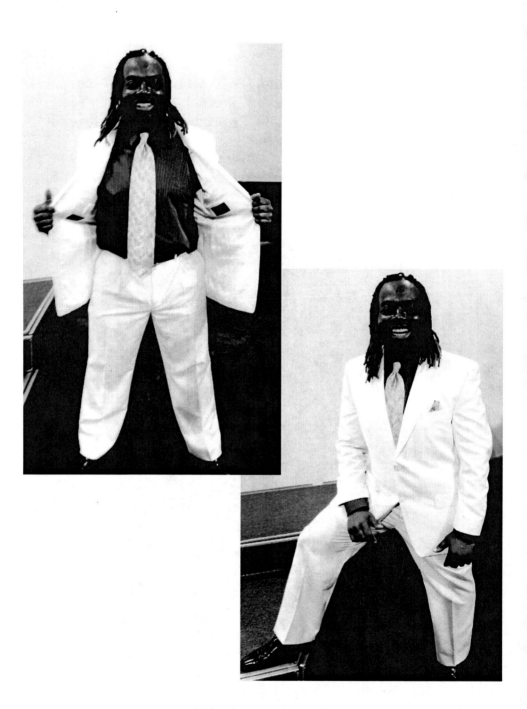

Reverend Charles Cooper July 17, 2011
A new man! A new life!

TESTIMONIALS

Before starting Ruben's program, my clothes didn't fit comfortably, my blood pressure was too high, my stamina too low, I didn't like the way my body looked in the mirror, I was concerned about my life expectancy, concerned over some physical and emotional areas that I want to be healed – and I couldn't SEE how to heal in any of those areas. I then made the decision to change. "When the student is ready, the teacher appears." That's when Ruben showed up. I discovered that I desired to be healthier more than I desired to not be. I also saw that I could release my old concerns about how long it was going to take to see/feel results – it's about the journey. My original physical goal was to have the healthy physical appearance that Ruben has (as close as I could with my body) by the end of the program. I also wanted to experience major steps forward in achieving visible/emotional/spiritual success over my concerns. My commitment was to follow the program faithfully. A goal is fine, but it also must contain the commitment, otherwise, forget the goal. The first day of class, the first actions I took were to get rid of all the foods in my home that aren't part of the program, and replaced them with foods that are. Next, I changed my exercise routine; increased my cardio with more walks, jogging, and small weights done to dancing CD's in my living room. I have made this whole program into a PLAY DATE. This is not work or drudgery, and I focus on the fun and the end results, not on where I am right now. Some of the results:

Physically: Clothes are fitting looser, wearing a suit I've not been able to get into for over 6 years, body looking slimmer, people noticing and commenting (how cool is that!), stamina up in all areas, blood pressure down.

Emotionally/Mentally: I feel the success, the determination, THE KNOWING, the patience, the joy, the willingness without the judgments of time or looks.

Spiritually: In my heart I see and know that I got the message at the right time because I've got a lot of personal accomplishments and exampling to do before I'm finished on the planet in this lifetime, and I am so very thankful for the time and energy to get at it. DO THIS PROGRAM!

- *John Early, Entrepreneur*

I had quit smoking a few months before attending. However, I was eating lots of sweets, sodas, junk food to replace my nicotine habit. My wife encouraged me to participate in this program. I wasn't sure I wanted to attend. I thought I would be forced to become a vegan, and I wasn't ready for that. She explained that the class was more about healthy living. What

I discovered in the program was how to create more energy with aerobic exercise, and how to feel better by eating more vegetables and fruits. I now exercise 5 days a week! I feel better in all areas – physically, emotionally, mentally and spiritually. I also noticed that when I don't exercise regularly, I have much less energy. So, that keeps me motivated to keep exercising!

- Harvey McDaniel, Insurance broker

Before the program, I wasn't sure about the most efficient way to maximize my exercising, and I ate meat and dairy. I decided to participate so I could learn information for myself and my clients. What I discovered from being in the program was the most efficient exercise program, and a food ladder that I agree with and could share with my clients. I then became vegan fully for six weeks, and am staying mostly vegetarian with occasional fish, and have been regularly exercising 5 – 6 days per week! As a result, I feel clearer spiritually and have increased my energy!!

– Brianna Mitchell, Holistic clinical hypnotherapist

I was aware of my poor health and physical state before the program, but I was unaware of the poor nutrition I had. I decided to participate because I had overheard part of the previous program and was impressed. Some of the key things

I learned were the unfathomable lies we are told by the food and beverage world and manufacturers. Subsequently, I became a vegan and increased my physical fitness program. As a result, I have lost 15 pounds, and feel like I am honest with myself for the first time around food. I have broken my addiction to sugar and it feels great!!

– Charlotte Parks, Licensed MFT - Therapist for Children

My goal was to exercise more regularly and eat healthier. I ate pretty healthy already, but I was irregular in my exercise. I chose to participate in this program because I wanted to know more about being healthy and I wanted to find strategies that would help me do more of what I needed. In the program, I learned why I had a hard time exercising consistently – my old blueprint was that adult women (my mother) did not exercise – what was important was to be thin and beautiful. I also gained a greater understanding about how my body works!! Subsequently, I decided to take responsibility for my exercise. I even worked out 6 days last week! I am really committed to exercising and getting even more healthy. I also gained the perspective of "living into possibility." As a result of being in this program, I am getting stronger physically, I feel good emotionally, I am mentally alert and spiritually connected!

- Kathy Fong, Wellness Coach, Sutter Health

Before the program I was confronted by lots of contradictory health and fitness information. I had experimented with lots of trial and error trying to sort things out. I decided to participate in this program because Ruben sounded like he knows what he's talking about, AND John Early vouched for him. I learned LOTS! Red Zone, eating every 3 hours, increasing mitochondria in cells through aerobic exercise, strength exercises, why are we drinking another species' milk, and especially why are adults drinking it? Glass of water in the morning, incline push-up, transformational principles reviewed, body-fat measurement. In fact, I was somewhat shocked by my percent body fat and what if should be! Subsequently, I began aerobic exercise 5-6 times a week. I quit drinking milk or using butter. I have water every morning and I do strength exercises. Because I quit dairy, I have stopped blowing my nose all the time. I have been consistently losing half to one pound of fat a week. When I went snowshoeing with my friends, I used to be in the middle or the back of the pack. Now, I'm way out in front and waiting for the others to catch up! How great is that!

- *Bob Vopacke, Retired controller, in his 60's*

I am recovering from cancer and all that it entails. Before I started this course, I was depressed, a couch potato, very weak and unbalanced. I was told by my doctor that at this age and weight, I would be stuck for the rest of my life. In Ruben's program, I learned that what I had perceived as an obstacle, truly believing it to be an impossibility – just isn't so! I have NEVER taken such a comprehensive, condensed health class that addresses ALL aspects of health – diet, exercise, stress, spirit – from a person of such great warmth, integrity, and who WALKS his talk! I learned specifics on nutrition and exercise to a whole different level. Ruben is not a "do as I say" kinda guy. He gives you the WHY of it all. He inspires you to feel joyful in the challenge and opportunity of living a life of great wellness. He is very clear and easy to follow. He uses multimedia, listening, reading, powerpoint, is very interactive... all types of learners will relate. He is an outstanding speaker and presenter! Funny, compassionate, total expert in his field, a very compelling and inspiring speaker. I now know that I will recover strength through daily exercise and a vegan lifestyle. I have given up meat and dairy. I meditate daily. I feel HOPEFUL now – dare I say CONFIDENT – that I CAN regain and improve my health following cancer. Some of my results so far are that my rosacea (which was really bad) has cleared. I have lost six pounds in six weeks. I have given up caffeine and sodas, and my urine is clear for the first time! I feel more alert and energetic than ever! This program is a MUST!!

- *Elisabeth Davis, writer*

Before I participated in this course I was unable to loose weight. I have been wanting to feel "light" for a very long time – years. I had also struggled with severe exercise-induced asthma for about ten years. As a registered nurse at Sutter, I thought I knew a lot about health and nutrition. In Ruben's course I discovered the many "myths" about food and exercise, and learned the "truths" of how the body truly works – based on the physiology and biochemistry of our human design. Ruben's presentation was excellent and well organized. He is clear, concise, motivational and REAL. I have now incorporated an entirely vegan food plan and have discovered exciting recipes! I plan to be more consistent with exercise, strength and cardio. As a result of being in the program, I have lost six pounds in seven weeks. I feel lighter! I have no more heartburn! I enjoy good food. And my breathing has improved substantially – I no longer have "asthma."

- Laraine Carver, RN for Sutter Health

ABOUT THE AUTHOR

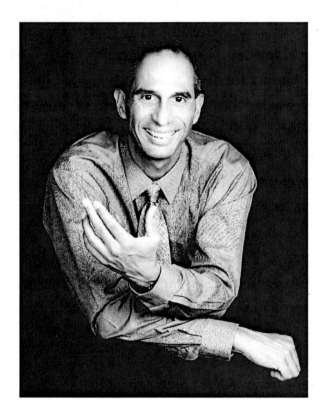

Award-winning speaker, Ruben J. Guzman, M.P.H. lives as proof of what he presents. In October 1990, he ruptured his achilles while playing basketball. Subsequently, he became apathetic about his health and gained weight. In January 1995, he began his transformation. Ruben personally lost over 50 pounds of fat and has been healthy and fit ever since. But more importantly, he has empowered hundreds to do the same for themselves. Ruben has conducted programs for various organizations including the California State Capitol,

City of Sacramento, Hewlett-Packard, VSP, Intel, Yahoo, UC Davis, Kaiser and Mercy Healthcare, the Los Angeles County Sheriffs, and several departments for the State. He is also an expert speaker for Vistage International, the world's largest CEO organization, and travels extensively training executives in health, leadership and communication. Coach Ruben works with CEOs, executives and organizations empowering them to create a thriving culture with dynamic leadership. A professor at DeVry University, Ruben teaches classes in leadership, communication and psychology. He holds a Masters degree in Public Health (MPH) from UCLA specializing in Behavioral Sciences and Health Promotion, and spent three years at UC Davis Medical School. He was a professional swimming coach for 30 years. Ruben is nationally certified as a personal trainer and nutrition consultant, and has successfully coached and trained many champions in sports, business and health. His dynamic energy is both inspirational and motivating!

Coach Ruben provides keynote addresses, workshops, corporate wellness programs, healthy lifestyle coaching, business and executive coaching, thriving culture set-ups and organizational culture makeovers.

Visit his website at www.CoachRuben.com
He can be contacted at CoachRuben@CoachRuben.com
(916) 484-7415

CPSIA information can be obtained at www.ICGtesting.com
Printed in the USA
LVOW05s0445240314

378591LV00009BA/121/P

MERCEDES LACKEY

is the *New York Times* bestselling author of the Heralds of Valdemar and A Tale of the Five Hundred Kingdoms series, plus several other series and stand-alone books. Mercedes has more than fifty books in print, and some of her foreign editions can be found in Russian, Czech, Polish, French, Italian and Japanese. She has collaborated with such luminaries as Marion Zimmer Bradley, Anne McCaffrey and Andre Norton. She lives in Oklahoma with her husband and frequent collaborator, Larry Dixon, and their flock of parrots.

TANITH LEE

was born in 1947, in England. Unable to read until she was almost eight, she began to write at the age of nine. To date she has published almost seventy novels, ten short-story collections and well over two hundred short stories. Lee has also written for BBC Radio and TV. Her work has won several awards, and has been translated into more than twenty languages. She is married to the writer/artist John Kaiine. Readers can find more information about Lee at www.TanithLee.com or www.daughterofthenight.com.

C.E. MURPHY

holds an utterly impractical degree in English and history. At age six, Catie submitted several poems to an elementary school publication. The teacher producing it chose (inevitably) the one Catie thought was the worst of the three, but he also stopped her in the hall one day and said two words that made an indelible impression: "Keep writing." It was sound advice, and she's pretty much never looked back. More information about Catie and her writing can be found at www.cemurphy.net.